DEFINITIONS OF BIOMATERIALS
FOR THE TWENTY-FIRST CENTURY

DEFINITIONS OF BIOMATERIALS FOR THE TWENTY-FIRST CENTURY

Proceedings of a Consensus Conference
Held in Chengdu, People's Republic of China
June 11th and 12th 2018

Organized under the auspices of the International Union of Societies for Biomaterials
Science & Engineering

Hosted and supported by Sichuan University, Chengdu and the Chinese
Society for Biomaterials, China

Proceedings edited by

PROFESSOR DAVID WILLIAMS
Wake Forest Institute of Regenerative Medicine, Winston-Salem, NC, United States

and

PROFESSOR XINGDONG ZHANG, PRESIDENT IUSBSE
Sichuan University, Chengdu, China
Conference on Definitions in Biomaterials 2018 Executive Committee:
James Anderson, Case Western Reserve University, Cleveland, OH, United States
Kristi Anseth, University of Colorado at Boulder, Boulder, CO, United States
Xiaobing Fu, General Hospital of PLA, Beijing, China
Kazunori Kataoka, University of Tokyo, Tokyo, Japan
Cato Laurencin, University of Connecticut, Hartford, CT, United States
Keith McLean, CSIRO, Melbourne, VIC, Australia
Nicholas Peppas, University of Texas at Austin, Austin, TX, United States
David Williams, Wake Forest Institute of Regenerative Medicine, Winston-Salem, NC, United States
Xingdong Zhang, Sichuan University, Chengdu, China

ELSEVIER

Elsevier
Radarweg 29, PO Box 211, 1000 AE Amsterdam, Netherlands
The Boulevard, Langford Lane, Kidlington, Oxford OX5 1GB, United Kingdom
50 Hampshire Street, 5th Floor, Cambridge, MA 02139, United States

Notices
Knowledge and best practice in this field are constantly changing. As new research and experience broaden our understanding, changes in research methods, professional practices, or medical treatment may become necessary.

Practitioners and researchers must always rely on their own experience and knowledge in evaluating and using any information, methods, compounds, or experiments described herein. In using such information or methods they should be mindful of their own safety and the safety of others, including parties for whom they have a professional responsibility.

To the fullest extent of the law, neither the Publisher nor the authors, contributors, or editors, assume any liability for any injury and/or damage to persons or property as a matter of products liability, negligence or otherwise, or from any use or operation of any methods, products, instructions, or ideas contained in the material herein.

British Library Cataloguing-in-Publication Data
A catalogue record for this book is available from the British Library

Library of Congress Cataloging-in-Publication Data
A catalog record for this book is available from the Library of Congress

ISBN: 978-0-12-818291-8

For Information on all Elsevier publications
visit our website at https://www.elsevier.com/books-and-journals

Publisher: Matthew Deans
Acquisition Editor: Sabrina Webber
Editorial Project Manager: Mariana L. Kuhl
Production Project Manager: Joy Christel Neumarin Honest Thangiah
Cover Designer: Christian J. Bilbow

Typeset by MPS Limited, Chennai, India

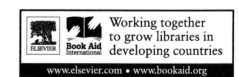
Working together
to grow libraries in
developing countries

www.elsevier.com • www.bookaid.org

Contents

Attendees at Chengdu Definitions in Biomaterials Conference 2019

Hua Ai   Sichuan University, Chengdu, China

James Anderson   Department Pathology, Case Western Reserve University, Cleveland, OH, United States

Kristi Anseth   Chemical and Biological Engineering, University of Colorado at Boulder, Boulder, CO, United States

Iulian Antoniac   University Politehnica of Bucharest, Bucharest, Romania

Mário Barbosa   i3S/INEB, University of Porto, Porto, Portugal

Bikramjit Basu   Materials Research Centre, Indian Institute of Sciences, Bangalore, India

Serena Best   Materials Science & Metallurgy, University of Cambridge, Cambridge, United Kingdom

Ruggero Bettini   Dipartimento di Scienze degli Alimenti e del Farmaco, University of Parma, Parma, Italy

Deon Bezuidenhout   Cardiothoracic Surgery, University of Cape Town, Cape Town, South Africa

Rena Bizios   Biomedical Engineering, University of Texas at San Antonio, San Antonio, TX, United States

John Brash   Biomedical Engineering, McMaster University, Hamilton, ON, Canada

Yilin Cao   Plastic Surgery, 9th People's Hospital, Shanghai Jiao Tong University, Shanghai, China

Jiang Chang   Biomaterials & Tissue Engineering Centre, Shanghai Institute of Ceramics, CAS, Shanghai, China

Guoping Chen   MANA, National Institute for Materials Science, Ibaraki, Japan

Elizabeth Cosgriff-Hernandez   Biomedical Engineering, University of Texas at Austin, Austin, TX, United States

Arthur Coury   Chemical Engineering, Northeastern University, Boston, MA, United States

Jiandong Ding   Department of Macromolecular Science, Jiangwan Campus of Fudan University, Shanghai, China

Xiaobing Fu   Molecular Cell Biology Laboratory, Chinese PLA General Hospital, Beijing, China

Andrés García   Mechanical Engineering, Georgia Institute of Technology, Atlanta, GA, United States

Brendan Harley   Chemical and Biomolecular Engineering, University of Illinois, Urbana, IL, United States

Jian Ji   Zhejiang University, Hangzhou, China

Kazunori Kataoka   Policy Alternatives Research Institute, University of Tokyo, Tokyo, Japan

Joachim Kohn   New Jersey Center for Biomaterials, Rutgers University, Piscataway, NJ, United States

Cato Laurencin Institute for Clinical and Translational Science, University of Connecticut, Farmington, CT, United States

Kam Leong Columbia University Department of Systems Biology, Irving Cancer Research Center, New York, NY, United States

Jui-Che Lin Chemical Engineering, National Cheng Kung University, Taipei, China

Changsheng Liu East China University of Science and Technology, Shanghai China

Helen Lu Biomedical Engineering, Columbia University, New York, NY, United States

Peter Ma Dentistry, University of Michigan, Ann Arbor, MI, United States

Keith McLean CSIRO, Parkville, VIC, Australia

Ling Qin Li Ka Shing Medical Sciences Building, Chinese University of Hong Kong, Prince of Wales Hospital, Shatin, New Territories Hong Kong, China

Ki-Dong Park Biomedical Engineering, Ajou University, Suwon, Korea

Nicholas Peppas Chemical Engineering, University of Texas at Austin, Austin, TX, United States

Laura Poole-Warren Biomedical Engineering, University of New South Wales, Sydney, NSW, Australia

Seeram Ramakrishna Center for Nanofibers & Nanotechnology, National University of Singapore, Singapore

John Ramshaw CSIRO, Parkville, VIC, Australia

Rui Reis Three Bs Laboratory, University of Minho, Guimarães, Portugal

Carl Simon Biomaterials Group, NIST, Gaithersburg, MD, United States

Wei Sun Mechanical Engineering, Drexel University, Philadelphia, PA, United States

Yasuhiko Tabata Biomaterials, Institute for Frontier Medical Sciences, Kyoto University, Kyoto, Japan

Madoka Takai Bioengineering, University of Tokyo, Tokyo, Japan

Timmie Topoleski Mechanical Engineering, University of Maryland, Baltimore, MD, United States

Maria J. Vicent CIPF, C/Eduardo Primo Yúfera, Valencia, Spain

William Wagner McGowan Institute for Regenerative Medicine, University of Pittsburgh, Pittsburgh, PA, United States

Yingjun Wang School of Materials Science and Engineering, South China University of Technology, Guangzhou, China

Yunbing Wang Sichuan University, Sichuan, China

David Williams Wake Forest Institute of Regenerative Medicine, Winston-Salem, NC, United States

Frank Witte Charité-Universitätsmedizin, Berlin-Brandenburg Center for Regenerative Therapies, Julius Wolff Institute, Berlin, Germany

Tingfei Xi Beijing Key Lab of Regenerative Medicine in Orthopedics, Chinese PLA General Hospital, Beijing, China

Hanry Yu Translational Mechanobiology Laboratory, National University of Singapore, Singapore

Kai Zhang Sichuan University, Sichuan, China

Xingdong Zhang Sichuan University, Sichuan, China

Yuliang Zhao National Center for Nanoscience and Technology, Beijing, China

Acknowledgments

This work and the conference were supported by the 111 Project (No. B16033). Thanks go to Sichuan University and the Chinese Society for Biomaterials for their support in hosting the conference. We would also like to thank Wanlu Zhao and his colleagues in the Sichuan University and the Chinese Society for Biomaterials for their efforts in organizing the conference and Peggy O'Donnell for her assistance in transcribing the proceedings.

I

Introduction

A Background

In March 1986, a consensus conference, organized under the auspices of the European Society of Biomaterials, was held in Chester, United Kingdom. The theme of the conference was "definitions in biomaterials"; the Proceedings were published in 1987 by Elsevier.[1]

In describing the objectives of the conference, the editor of those proceedings drew attention to situations where new scientific or technical subjects develop, partly as spin-offs from established disciplines and partly as initiatives driven by scientific or market forces, in which new words and syntax, often with characteristics of jargon or scientific inconsistency, tend to emerge. Some of these words and phrases rapidly become assimilated into common language while others are retained within the language of the professionals.

It was proposed that biomaterials science was one of those areas of advanced technology where a large number of new terms were being introduced or invented. Controversy was increasing over the use of these terms. Some of them were words that had been derived within an established area but were now being used in the biomaterials context with a different meaning. In other situations, there was a clear need for a new word to describe a phenomenon or object, where there was no acceptable existing word, but the emergence of the descriptive word or phrase did not follow etymological reasoning, or indeed, common sense. Part of the problem lay within the multi- and interdisciplinary nature of the subject, as pathologists tried to describe corrosion mechanisms within metallic devices and metallurgists tried to describe inflammatory responses.

Whatever the cause of the laxity of definitions and of their undisciplined use, the results are the same: confusion about the subject under discussion, ambiguity in the literature, and dangerous or misleading uncertainties in the promulgation of knowledge. Research, education, and clinical uses all suffer.

At the 1986 conference, terms were discussed under four areas: general biomaterials, blood compatibility, general biocompatibility, and interfacial activity. These were dealt within four sessions, for each of which there was a moderator and a reporter. The reporter assembled a list of definitions that emerged within that session and put preferred

---

[1] Williams D F, (ed.) *Definitions in Biomaterials*, Progress in Biomedical Engineering, Vol 4, Elsevier: Amsterdam, 1987.

definitions to a vote; a definition was considered to have achieved consensus if no less than 75% of those present voted in favor.

A summary of terms that achieved consensus, and those that were discussed but did not gain consensus, is found in Box I.

BOX I

Summary of Definitions Produced in the 1986 Meeting

The Conference Chair/Proceedings Editor (David Williams), together with session Moderators and Reporters, produced lists (in alphabetical order) of definitions that achieved consensus, those that were discussed that reached provisional agreement but without consensus at that time, those that were discussed but did not achieve any agreement or consensus, and those that were discussed but where delegates agreed that there was no need for such a term, its use therefore being deprecated.

DEFINITIONS WITH CONSENSUS

Artificial Organ
A medical device that replaces, in part or in whole, the function of one of the organs of the body

Bioactive Material
A material which has been designed to induce specific biological activity

Bioadhesion
The adhesion of cells and/or tissues to the surface of a material

Bioattachment
The fastening of cells and/or tissue to the surface of a material, including mechanical interlocking

Biocompatibility
The ability of a material to perform with an appropriate host response in a specific application

Biomaterial
A nonviable material used in a medical device, intended to interact with biological systems

Bioprosthesis
An implantable prosthesis that consists totally or substantially, of nonviable, treated, donor tissue

Host Response
The reaction of a living system to the presence of a material

---

BOX I   (cont'd)

Hybrid Artificial Organ
    An artificial organ that is a combination of viable cells and one or more biomaterials

Implant
    A medical device made from one or more biomaterials that is intentionally placed within the body, either totally or partially buried beneath an epithelial surface

Medical Device
    An instrument, apparatus, implement, machine, contrivance, in vitro reagent, or other similar or related article, including any component, part or accessory, which is intended for use in the diagnosis of disease or other conditions, or in the cure, mitigation, treatment or prevention of disease in man

Prosthesis
    A device that replaces a limb, organ or tissue of the body

Thrombogenicity
    The property of a material which induces and/or promotes the formation of a thrombus

PROVISIONAL DEFINITIONS

Biodegradation
    The gradual breakdown of a material mediated by specific biological activity

Bioresorption
    The process of removal by cellular activity and/or dissolution of a material in a biological environment

Graft
    A piece of viable tissue or collection of viable cells transferred from a donor site to a recipient site for the purpose of reconstruction of the recipient site

Percutaneous Device
    A medical device that passes through the skin, remaining in that position for a significant length of time

Permucosal Device
    A medical device that passes through a mucosal surface, remaining in that position for a significant length of time

Transplant
    A complete structure, such as an organ, that is transferred from a site in a donor to a site in a recipient for the purpose of reconstruction of the recipient site

---

BOX I   (*cont'd*)

DEFINITION WITHOUT CONSENSUS

Foreign Body Reaction
    A variation in normal tissue behavior caused by the presence of a foreign material

TERMS TO BE DEPRECATED

Antithrombogenic
Biocompatible
Bioinert
Biological Performance
Biometal
Biopolymer
Biostability
Blood Compatibility
Material Rejection
Material Response
Thromboresistant

It is now over 30 years since these definitions were formulated and agreed. Some appear to have stood the test of time; the definition of biocompatibility, for example, is still very widely used and has not been superseded.[2] Many other definitions that achieved consensus, however, are clearly in need of a fresh look, partly as a result of much greater clarity on the scientific and clinical issues involved and partly because biomaterials science has expanded in scope,[3] so that it encompasses far more than implantable devices, which were the main focus in the 1980s. It is now necessary to consider the meaning of terms used within the context of the applications of materials in regenerative medicine/tissue engineering, drug, vaccine, and gene delivery and diagnostic procedures using biomaterial-based agents. The 2018 definitions conference in Chengdu was organized in order to address these issues.

B Logistics of the Consensus Conference

There were some similarities between the procedural aspects of the 1986 and 2018 conferences. The idea to hold the latter was originated in May 2016 during the 10th World Biomaterials Congress at Montreal, Canada, where Professor Xingdong Zhang, President of IUSBSE, met and exchanged thoughts with James Anderson, Kam Leong, Nicholas

[2] Williams D F, On the mechanisms of biocompatibility, *Biomaterials* 2008; 29:2941-53.

[3] Williams D F, On the nature of biomaterials, *Biomaterials* 2009; 30:5897-909.

Peppas, Buddy Ratner, William Wagner, David Williams, and many other leaders in the field, who enthusiastically supported the idea.

Xingdong Zhang met with David Williams for an initial planning meeting in Chengdu in May 2017 and with Nicholas Peppas in late August before he officially proposed the 2018 conference to the IUSBSE, which was unanimously approved at the 2017 annual meeting of IUSBSE on September 4th, 2017. In mid-September 2017, Zhang reported to the President of Sichuan University and recommended hosting and sponsoring this important conference, which was later approved. An Executive Committee was established through discussion with some experts in this field, and the recommendations arising from the early preparation meetings were presented to the Executive Committee. Representative members met in Chengdu in January 2018. It was agreed that the meeting would have six subject-specific sessions, dealing with General Biomaterials, Biocompatibility, Drugs and Genes Delivery, Implantable and Interventional Devices, Regenerative Medicine, and Emerging Biomaterials and Technologies. Each session would have a plenary speaker, who would present the preferred options for definitions of, typically, 15 terms. Each session would have a moderator who would chair the discussions about these terms, and a reporter, who would prepare the list of definitions preferred by delegates (which could be consistent with the recommendation of the plenary speaker, or a modified version of that definition, or indeed any definition proposed by any delegate) and take and record the votes. *It was agreed that at least 75% of those present would need to approve a proposed definition for it to be deemed to have achieved consensus; furthermore, a minimum of 30 people voting in the affirmative was necessary to confirm consensus to take into account those who abstained or were absent. It was also agreed that a definition that received a vote of 50%—74% would be deemed to have provisional consensus.* As a final point, since most discussions concentrated on scientific content, and time was very limited for discussion of syntax, a few definitions appeared to have less-than-ideal grammatical structure when the vote was taken. The editor, David Williams, was given authority to make minor adjustments to the wording, with the caveat that any such changes would be brought to the attention of delegates during the approval process of these Proceedings.

The schedule of plenary speakers, moderators, and reporters were agreed as follows:

Session	Plenary Speaker	Moderator	Reporter
General biomaterials	David Williams	Kai Zhang	Carl Simon
Biocompatibility	James Anderson	Andrés García	Serena Best
Drugs and genes delivery	Nicholas Peppas	Kazunori Kataoka	Maria J. Vicent
Implantable and interventional devices	Jiang Chang	Arthur Coury	Keith McLean
Regenerative medicine	William Wagner	Cato Laurencin	Helen Lu
Emerging biomaterials and technologies	Kristi Anseth	Kam Leong	Jiandong Ding

The initial intention was that the speaker would present for discussion one or more potential definitions for each term, using slides as appropriate, and the major part of each 2-hour session would be taken up in discussion, leading to rejection of some options and, if necessary, modification of the preferred definitions, with a final vote, recorded electroni-cally and anonymously. The pattern of presentation/discussion did vary from session to session and by no means all the offered terms and definitions were discussed, in view of time constraints.

A final session had been scheduled for the afternoon of the second day for summary discussions; in practice, this was used to return to some definitions that required more time for finalization and to include some other terms that delegates considered should have been included.

The discussions at the meeting were recorded, and a transcript of the whole conference was constructed by David Williams and Peggy O'Donnell. These Proceedings are based on that transcript, being edited by David Williams and Xingdong Zhang. Draft proceed-ings were submitted, first to the Executive Committee and then to all delegates, for approval prior to publication.

C Structure of Definitions

It is not possible, and indeed it would be unwise to try, to definitively prescribe the structure of definitions to be included in any dictionary or encyclopedia. However, when the purpose of a collection of definitions is to improve the clarity of a language dealing with a specific subject, it is helpful for the definitions to have some consistency in struc-ture and form. A few general principles were provided to the delegates in advance of the meeting, as follows:

- In many situations, the term to be defined is also used in general or scientific contexts: definitions of these terms in the biomaterial context should not be inconsistent with the more general meanings but may be amplified in order to emphasize that context.
- The definition should not include the word that is being defined. Note that in some composite terms (e.g., metallic biomaterial), this cannot be avoided.
- The definition should not include examples (avoid "e.g.," "such as," "including").
- The definition should not normally provide details of mechanisms.
- The definition should not include vague, imprecise, or generic phrases, such as "x is the field of..." or "y is the science of...."
- The definition should not necessarily be the same as any definition used for regulatory, testing protocol, or standards purposes, but may take them into account.
- Note that some definitions are conceptual in nature (such as the 1986 definition of "biocompatibility"), while others are operational (such as the 1986 definition of "implant"). Both are valid and have their own uses and merits.

D Introductory General Definitions

Some very basic terms are used within definitions; it is helpful to have a clear under-standing of what each of these terms mean to avoid confusion. The following suggestions for basic definitions, in some cases with multiple options, were provided for the delegates.

Material

A substance useful for making objects[4]

Device

Something contrived for a specific purpose[4]
or
Something made or adapted for a particular purpose

Drug

Any substance, natural or synthetic, which has a physiological action on a living body, either when used for the treatment of disease, or the alleviation of pain, or for self-indulgence or recreation[4]
or
A substance intended for use in the diagnosis, cure, mitigation, treatment or prevention of disease: a substance (other than food) intended to affect the structure or any function of the body[5]

Organ

Part of a body adapted and specialized for the performance of a particular function

Tissue

A level of organization in multicellular organisms consisting of a group of structurally and functionally similar cells and their intercellular material[6]

Degradation

Deleterious change in the chemical structure, physical properties or appearance of a material[4]
or
An irreversible process leading to a change of the structure of a material, characterized by a loss of properties and/or fragmentation

Resorption

The breakdown of a structure and consequent assimilation of resulting components into their environment

Absorption

The process of taking some agent into a substance by chemical or physical action

Nanoscale

Having one or more dimensions of the order of 100 nm or less

[4] Williams D F, The Williams Dictionary of Biomaterials, Liverpool University Press, 1999, Liverpool.

[5] US Food & Drugs Administration, Drugs@ FDA Glossary.

[6] Encyclopedia Britannica.

Immunity

The capacity of a body to recognize the intrusion of foreign material and to mobilize cells and cell products to effectively remove that material

Mesh

An open fabric made of intertwined fibers

Vector

A carrier that transfers a biological substance, especially an infective agent, from one site to another

E Terms to be Discussed

Members of the Executive Committee who met in Chengdu in January 2018 were provided with a provisional list of terms that could be discussed and defined at the Consensus Conference. This list was amended during the January meeting and refined over the following months. The provisional list, along with suggestions of the Editor, David Williams, for possible definitions, is provided in Annex A.

F Structure of the Proceedings

The sessions were arranged on the basis of terms within reasonably well-contained groups, recognizing that there was likely to be some overlap. The identity of these sessions and their content became less clear over time, and some terms had relevance to, and were considered in, more than one session. These Proceedings have therefore been organized with a hierarchical rather than session-based structure. The outline of this structure is shown in Fig. 1.1.

By way of example, the first term to be discussed and defined was biomaterial, and its putative synonym biomedical material. There are then seven groups of related terms: subsets

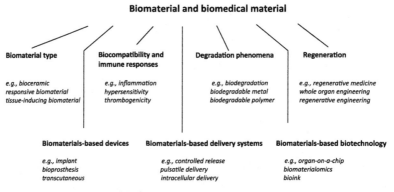

FIGURE 1.1 Hierarchical Structure of Definitions.

of biomaterial, biocompatibility and immune responses, degradation phenomena, regeneration, biomaterial-based devices, biomaterial-based delivery systems, and biomaterials-based biotechnology.

For each session, the plenary speakers were asked to prepare suggested definitions for a group of terms, previously agreed with the Executive Committee, such lists being included in the Final Program made available to all delegates. In most cases, it became clear, because of the volume and intensity of discussions, that there would be insufficient time for complete review of all tabled terms, and speakers were invited to prioritize the words for discussion.

In each section of these Proceedings, all relevant terms slated for examination are included. For each word/term, the following information is provided:

- The term, together with any suggested synonym,
- The preliminary definition(s) suggested before the conference, as indicated in Annex A,
- The definition(s) suggested by the Plenary Speaker, together with any text used to explain or justify the choices,
- An edited version of the discussions. It should be noted that both video and audio recordings were made of all sessions. A full transcript of all audio recordings was made by David Williams and the editorial assistant Peggy O'Donnell, with the help of a professional transcription service. David Williams then extracted all conversations, from one or more sessions, relevant to each term and constructed the edited version of each discussion,
- The final definition(s) produced for each term,
- The result of the vote,
- Any subsequent commentary about the definition.

In each section, the terms are generally discussed in the order; those which received consensus, terms which achieved provisional consensus, terms discussed and voted but without consensus and words included in the agenda but not discussed. Occasionally, logic has suggested that this order should not be followed, especially when a term that was not voted on is highly relevant to one that did achieve consensus, so that they should be discussed together.

As a final point on the structure and format of these Proceedings, the editors have made every effort to accurately reflect all of the contributions. Bearing in mind many of the delegates did not have English as their first language, there were inevitably several situations in which a contribution could not be fully transcribed. This effect was exaggerated by some delegates failing to speak into their microphones on every occasion, where multiple delegates spoke at the same time, or when there was excessive cross-talk. David Williams and Peggy O'Donnell have separately and collectively reviewed, and re-reviewed, difficult sections, and have used the context of the discussion, to produce the best options for statements. The editors have also tried to produce the best syntax through the elimination of repetitive or idiosyncratic phrases where it was possible to do so without losing meaning. Because so many of the delegates refer to individual words or phrases that are contained in definitions under discussion, liberal use has been made of parentheses in an attempt to avoid grammatical confusion.

G Introductory Comments at the Conference

The following is an edited version of the introductory comments made to the conference delegates.

Xingdong Zhang	Dear colleagues, good morning. Welcome to the Consensus Conference of Biomaterial Definitions. The definition of biomaterials standardizes the connotation of the discipline for biomaterial science and engineering, and it is very important for biomaterials development. There are 53 outstanding biomaterial experts from 17 countries and regions. The conference is organized under the auspices of the International Union of Society for Biomaterial Science Engineering. I believe it will be a big success, and become a certain milestone event in the development of biomaterials.
Xingdong Zhang	This conference is hosted by Sichuan University and the Chinese Society of Biomaterials. Professor Fu is the President of the Chinese Society of Biomaterials and Dr. Keith McLean is the Secretary of the IUSBSE. Now I would like to recognize Professor Williams.
David Williams	I will be chairing the first session this morning. At the beginning of my presentation, I will go through the procedures we're going to adopt here today. You have received documents from me over the last few months. We had several meetings yesterday to try to refine these, so I will try very briefly to let you know exactly how it is going to happen today.
David Williams	Thank you Professor Zhang for hosting us here in Chengdu, and for providing the sponsorship for this meeting. I remind you all that this is an immensely important meeting, and I would like everybody to recognize how important it is that you stay in the room, participate in the discussions, and participate in the votes.
David Williams	As normal, you would declare any conflict of interest in a presentation. Right now, I declare I have no conflict of interest as far as definitions are concern, except as you'd have heard, I organized, chaired, and was editor of the first set of definitions, the definition conference back in 1986 in Chester in UK. I do not mind if any of our definitions then are changed at this meeting, as part of the rationale of us being here. So, I have no real conflict of interest there.
David Williams	There are six sessions, as you have seen in the program. Each session has a plenary speaker, a moderator, and a reporter. Those three people will sit at this end of this table during the presentations. The plenary speaker presents the definitions that they want to use, preferably with a little rationale of why they're choosing those.

David Williams	The moderator will chair the discussion. I emphasize that I would like everybody to think carefully and contribute to that discussion where appropriate. The whole program is being recorded, and I will be transcribing the whole recording. It will be helpful to have recognition of the name of the speaker.
David Williams	The reporter will be taking notes during this time, and at the end we will have voting. We will conduct a vote on the position of all the delegates here with respect to each term. I emphasize it is good we all stay in the room throughout.
David Williams	You will vote either "yes," meaning you agree with the definition or "no," you do not agree. Or you may abstain. "Yes" means you completely agree with the definition which is up for voting. We had a good discussion about what "no" means yesterday. Primarily it means "No, you do not agree," or you have some real problem with the wording of the definition. You simply do not agree for that term to have consensus.
David Williams	"Abstain" means you have no view either way, which really means that it may be out of your field, or the speaker and the discussion has not persuaded you which side to go. I emphasize we want abstentions to be at a minimum, so we can achieve as good a consensus as possible.
David Williams	To get consensus, we need 75% or more "yes" votes. That is quite high. We want our position to have authority and credibility and that is why I suggested going this high. However, if there are too many abstentions, it will mean that 75% was not actually a good number. And so, we put in another criteria: 75% or more "yes" votes, and a minimum of 30 votes in total to give consensus.
David Williams	If the vote means that there are between 50% and 74%, that will give us provisional consensus. Back in the Chester conference, quite a few terms were discussed. In some cases there was fairly general agreement but not good enough for consensus, thus the terms were deemed to have provisional consensus. Now some of them have moved forward to be considered further.
David Williams	With less than 50%, there is no consensus, and that will be recorded. Similarly, terms presented by some of the speakers where there's no time for discussion, and no vote taken, those will also be recorded, but it will say "No vote taken."
David Williams	We have a final session tomorrow afternoon. I emphasize this is not a time to try to rehash the discussion, and trying to change the vote in your favor. That's not what we're trying to do tomorrow afternoon. There may be some areas where we need clarity, where there may be inconsistencies between terms defined in different sessions.

David Williams	The proceedings of the conference will be published as Professor Zhang has mentioned by Elsevier. I and Peggy O'Donnell will be transcribing these, and within one month, I will have a version of that sent to Professor Zhang. I emphasize here that during the meeting, or within a few days of the meeting, if you have any comment to make to me which you'd like me to take into account, please send me by email. I cannot guarantee to take them into account, but I will look at it very carefully. But it has to be done in short order.
David Williams	As soon as Professor Zhang has seen my draft, he will give it to the Executive Committee members, and the plenary speakers, for them to make any comment. Again, not to go back to argue again, but to look for accuracy and consistency. The next draft will go to everybody in this room. Within a few days, we will require you to make any comments, again emphasizing we do not wish you to go over everything again, but let me know of anything which you see as a glaring omission, or some deficiency on my behalf.
David Williams	Hopefully Elsevier will have everything in their office by the end of September, and probably they will publish it early next year. Obviously, we would like this to be done as soon as possible.
David Williams	The last point there, I refer to as the Chengdu Declaration. This is potentially very important. We will discuss it in more detail tomorrow afternoon. Let me just emphasize the importance of this. We hope that the definitions that achieve consensus here will be recognized by the biomaterials community for years to come and will be the preferred definitions that they use. One way we can do this is collectively for us to sign a declaration saying, "We believe we have achieved consensus with these definitions and urge all people to use them as appropriate." If we agree, we will ask the editors and publishers of the major journals to include this as a note in their journal.
David Williams	One important rationale for this is that Elsevier initially asked us to have a copyright agreement for everybody in the room. I strongly argued against that. I see no value to anybody in the room for doing that. Professor Zhang and I will sign a copyright agreement. But for anybody signing the copyright agreement, it would mean they could not say anywhere else what they said, which is recorded here. I did not want to do that.
David Williams	On the other hand, we needed to give recognition to everybody in the room. You have come a long way. You are a very important part of this. This Declaration will state all the names of people here, so they can say, "I was part of that." And that is now part of the record. I will give you more the rationale of that as we go through tomorrow.

David Williams	That's the procedures. Before I start on the general biomaterial session, just let me make a note about what I referred to as the structure of definitions. I am not going to great detail here. In the notes you have, on page 90, you will find my summary of these issues. I cannot and would not even try to tell plenary speakers how to construct their definition. That is entirely up to them. But there are some ground rules I would like us to consider, and I think there are important issues here. When you look at good, proper dictionaries, there is usually some sort of structure.
David Williams	First of all, the terms to be defined may also be used in general scientific context. We always have to bear that in mind, although sometimes our definitions should just add the biomedical context to that general discussion.
David Williams	A definition should not include the word that is being defined. In other words, with a definition of the word "biomaterial," which is the heading, we do not start by saying, "A biomaterial is." That is already implied. Sometimes you cannot avoid this, especially with terms that include multiple words: we will see a few of those.
David Williams	It is my preference the definitions should not include examples. A definition should not say, "For example," or "including" or things like that. Sometimes you cannot avoid it, but that is certainly the preference.
David Williams	The definition should not normally provide details of mechanisms. That is for other publications. Again, sometimes that cannot be avoided, but it is preferred that we do not do that.
David Williams	The definition should not include vague, imprecise, or generic phrases, such as, "X is the field of," or "Y is the science of." That maybe a contentious issue. I will refer you to the original definition of tissue engineering by Bob Langer and Jay Vacanti; it starts with "Tissue engineering is an interdisciplinary field that applies, etc." That was very good at the time and it pointed the way for tissue engineering, but that to me is not a good definition starting off with "an interdisciplinary field."
David Williams	The definition should not necessarily be the same as that used for regulatory, testing protocols, or standard procedures, but may take them into account. That is very important. We know, for example, the FDA has many definitions, and they are there for all to determine how these terms are defined within the regulatory context. I can perfectly understand that. But that is not necessarily scientifically based. It's legally based, or procedurally based, and it is not necessary for us to do that.
David Williams	And my final note there is that some definitions are conceptual in nature. For example, with the Chester definition of "biocompatibility." You will see that it is a concept. Others are

	operational, for example the definition, back in 1986, of "implant." Both are valid, and I do not have any preference for either. We will use these on their own merits.
David Williams	I should also add that there are some terms, some basic words, which we will find in many of our definitions. But these are general definitions. I am not going through the details now; you can see these on page 91-92 of the book. If anybody looking at these basic, generic definitions has any problems, let me know and we can discuss them tomorrow afternoon. I do not believe anything is contentious here.
Xingdong Zhang	Are there any questions about the conference, the procedure and rules, and the proceedings and the timeline?
Nicholas Peppas	I move that the procedures be approved as presented by David Williams. Thank you.
David Williams	Thank you Professor Zhang. Also, Professor Zhang asked me if I would include somewhere the definitions that achieved consensus way back in 1986. Those are in the booklet, page 120-121.
David Williams	Now, there are many people in the room, who we already know, do not agree with everything. It is a potentially contentious subject area. And for example, my good friend Jim Anderson here. He and I, I believe, were the only people in this room who attended the Chester meeting. We've had our arguments for 40 odd years. Sometimes we agree, sometimes we do not agree. Nearly always, Jim, I think I can say, we end up in friendship. That's very, very important for today's presentation.

Editor's Note: The Chengdu Declaration mentioned in this section is given in Annex B.

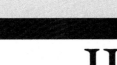

II

Biomaterials and biomedical materials

Discussed in Session I
Session I Plenary Presentation: *David Williams*
Session I Moderator: *Kai Zhang*
Session I Reporter: *Carl Simon*

Naturally, the most fundamental term to be discussed is that of "biomaterial" itself. This was considered alongside "biomedical material" in an attempt to determine whether these were synonymous or whether there was some subtle difference.

A Biomaterial

(a) Possible Definitions of "Biomaterial" Included in Final Program

1. A nonviable material used in a medical device, intended to interact with biological systems; *Definition that achieved consensus in Chester 1986*
2. Any matter, surface, or construct that interacts with biological systems[1]
3. A material intended to interface with biological systems to evaluate, treat, augment or replace any tissue, organ, or function of the body
4. A substance that has been engineered to take a form which, alone or part of a complex system, is used to direct, by control of interactions with components of living systems, the course of any therapeutic or diagnostic procedure, in human or veterinary medicine

(b) David Williams; Perspectives on "Biomaterial" and Suggested Definition

David Williams presented the four options given above, together with a simplified version of (4), as follows:

5. A substance that has been engineered to take a form which can direct, by control of interactions with living systems, the course of any therapeutic or diagnostic procedure

[1] National Institute of Biomedical Imaging and Bioengineering (USA: NIH).

In deciding on his recommendation, he drew attention to the fact that although the first definition above did achieve consensus in 1986, the extension of applications of biomaterials to situations other than conventional medical devices, and the doubtful validity of descriptors such as "nonviable," suggested that this definition was probably no longer valid. The second possibility is an example of a broader definition found in some glossaries. However, it does not specify medical applications and appears too imprecise to have any value in the present context. The third suggestion appeared in his own 1999 dictionary of biomaterials, but he suggested that it was too cumbersome now and too much resembled an FDA type definition with the emphasis on specific applications.

Option (4) was included in an essay on the nature of biomaterials published by Williams in 2009. He considered it to be still valid, being factually correct, but perhaps it was too long. He also pointed out that definition referred to both human and veterinary applications, the latter gaining increasing emphasis in clinical practice; however, if this phrase was included in this definition it would have to be included in many others and probably was not sufficiently important for this to be done.

(c) Edited Discussion of "Biomaterial"

In view of the above considerations, David Williams suggested that the more concise derivative of (4) was the best and proposed that this should be considered for consensus voting. Thus, the proposed definition of "Biomaterial" was:

A substance that has been engineered to take a form which can direct, by control of interactions with living systems, the course of any therapeutic or diagnostic procedure

Rena Bizios	I like the choices of the two terms: biomaterials and biomedical biomaterials. The first one is broader, and the second one is more specific. . .the first includes in my reading the composites, that we have a lot of composites in biomedical application. I am flattered because you used the term "engineer," but a lot of the new materials that I am familiar with are the result of scientists. And I do not want them to be alienated by the concept that only engineers that put together these materials. Thank you.
David Williams	Thank you Rena. I do not imply any real differences between engineers and scientists here, so I am not deprecating scientists here. I like the phrase "to engineer." I wrote a paper a number years ago, that was called "to engineer is to create," that was where the word "engineer" comes from. But I think that a scientist can do that as well as an engineer. If anybody wants to add that, I would be quite happy.
Nicholas Peppas	Congratulations David, this is a magnificent presentation, I wish all of them will be as detailed as this. I want to make a comment about "biomaterials," however, because you capture something that is happening in our field that is of concern to me. Other societies and other organizations, as you said, agricultural, and other organizations, have basically captured the term

"biomaterials" to describe the area that would include their interest and would make them workers and players in the field. I have a continuous fight with the American Institute of Chemical Engineers staff and members who want to use the word "biomaterials" to describe corn stalks and other substances to make ethanol. I think this body should express a very strong view about what we feel are biomaterials, and I hope that we will ask these organizations, such as the agricultural societies, to use alternative terminology. Thank you.

David Williams	Thank you, Nicholas. Very helpful. Obviously, that is not for a vote. But I will be very interested to see if any consensus view here to support what you said and I am very happy to include it in the proceedings. Does anybody have any comments on this, the other uses of the word biomaterials in the medical context? Is there anyone who does not agree with what Nick just said?
Laura Poole-Warren	I think that number five is coming closer to what we should be using; it is probably a little too wordy. It somewhat tautological to say "to take the form of" perhaps we can just say a substance or even a material that has been engineered to...etc. rather than to take the form.
David Williams	I have written it this way because, if you think back to my definition of a material, which is a substance used for making objects, it has to have form. I start this way because I cannot start by saying it is a material, a substance has been engineered to take a form. In other words, that substance now has a form, it is not just a gas, a fluid, or a solid.
Kai Zhang	Why can't you just use a material? A "material that can direct" instead of substance?
Laura Poole-Warren	So a material that has been engineered to control interactions with living systems. Something along those lines.
Arthur Coury	I have also taken a position in my definitions of biomaterial that it does have a form, it is a structure, so a saline solution is a synthetic solution, but it really doesn't have a structure, and so I agree that a form is another good word for structure.
Joachim Kohn	David, over the last 20 years, people have repeatedly made a comment about your definition of biomaterials, in the sense that it is a functional definition. It does not tell us what the biomaterial is; it only tells us what the biomaterial does. And that was perceived as a weakness of the definition. And I see that many of your definitions that you put forward now for biomaterials follow in that same trend. I personally have no objection to it, don't misunderstand me, but I wanted to point out that a definition usually defines what the material is, not defines a material by what it does.

David Williams   Yes. Joachim, that is a very good point. I did consider that some time ago and wasn't sure how to handle that because of the wide variety of materials that are used as biomaterials. So, I don't think we can define or characterize further any particular feature of a biomaterial in that sense for example, we are not saying it is a material which is metallic or polymeric, or ceramic, or composite; and it becomes too difficult and cumbersome to say it could be any of the above. I believe we are talking of biomaterials in the broad context of materials. I take your point. I don't know how to handle that any better.

Brendan Harley   I appreciate that in the definition of biomaterial that there is an action, maybe different from what Joachim was saying, because I have taken to now being asked to review a lot of biomaterial papers that are leaning to cellulose and other such materials. I think one thing that could set us apart is that our material, the biomaterial, that is designed for an action in the context of medical device. I think that may be one way by which we could have a strong definition of what we think biomaterials are.

David Williams   Thank you, Brendan. I think that is very helpful. The only issue I have with your first comment is that we end up with a definition which gets into mechanisms. That is what I have tried to say; it is a problem we often have, especially as we do not know all the mechanisms at this point. If we are very specific to one or two mechanisms, then we become self-limiting.

Mario Barbosa   This is about the beginning and the end of the list of definitions. I have difficulties in distinguishing between biomaterial, biological material, and biomedical material. If you use the definition of biomaterial, based on the application, to me biomedical material is more or less synonymous. The other thing I notice is that there is probably another term which we should use, which is biological material. Of course, wood is a biological material; bone and skin are biological materials, so maybe tomorrow this idea of introducing new terms could be raised again. I believe that the term "biological material" is needed somewhere.

David Williams   Thank you. I think that might be worth discussing. I think you are absolutely right, Mario; we have to be very clear what the difference is. That is why I was trying to say that the prefix "bio" can either mean "living" or "related to medical." I think we have to be very clear when we use those.

Andrés García   David, I like definition five better than the other ones simply because it is cleaner and reflects some of the ongoing work. Just a general suggestion; I am a little concerned about the word, or the phrase "by control of interactions with living systems." You could

	argue that there are many cases in which there is no designed control, so potentially just simply say, "through interactions with living systems" to remove "control."
David Williams	Good point, Andrés. I was trying to be very forward looking, then. You know what the intention is, but I accept your point.
Xiaobing Fu	Why do you emphasize "engineered," because there are some natural materials that are also biomaterials, such as when we treat burns we use skin from pigs. It is not engineered, but it is a biomaterial. So, why do you emphasize "engineered?"
David Williams	I mentioned before why we're talking about engineering, because with the vast majority of biomaterials in clinical applications, they are specifically arranged or created to have their function — that's why I used the word "engineer."
Nicholas Peppas	I have an alternative explanation. I think the problem, David, is because the word "engineer," as we use it in Europe and the United States, in plain English, means "to design." I don't think people appreciate that. So maybe, you might consider wordsmithing it and put the word "design" in parentheses, or you know … People are getting afraid when they hear the word "engineer." We use this term in the United States all the time.
David Williams	That's a very good point. I will be happy to remove "engineered" and say "designed." Okay?
Nicholas Peppas	Good.
Joachim Kohn	While we are waiting, can I make a comment about the number five for "biomaterials?" Okay, so I actually disagree with Andrés. I think this is the worst definition of all that are out there. Before we go there, I would like to make sure that they understand it. It's the most complex one. It includes within the definition several terms that need to be defined again, like "interaction," "living system," and so I think it is the one that is the most convoluted and most difficult to understand by people outside of the field. I think that David, you said that definitions should be simple, self-contained and easily understandable, and that is not what I would call definition number five. Thank you for considering this.
Kai Zhang	Do you have an alternative?
Joachim Kohn	Yes. I was asked if I have an alternative. Any of the one or two I think are simpler, and can be more readily used. We can more readily reach consensus around those than number five.
William Wagner	I think the problem with number five, is it is in our dreams. We would exclude 95% of biomaterials by that definition such as Dacron, and ePTFE. Just go down the list of things that are well-recognized as biomaterials today. We have no idea how we are controlling anything or any biological interaction. Is it protein

	adsorption and the response to that? I think that is a flaw with that definition that has to be changed.
Kai Zhang	Any other comments on number five? Definition number five for biomaterial?
Rena Bizios	Someone brought a comment regarding the word "control." Did we decide how this would be included, or not included, or substituted by another word?
Kai Zhang	Yes, let's work to modify this based from the number five definition of biomaterials. It feels to me that it's the most focused definition during the discussion.
David Williams	I have changed "engineered" to "designed." I think that met with approval. I am still trying to hear what the change by control of interactions. Was there a suggestion there? Maybe It should be changed to "through interactions."
Elizabeth Cosgriff-H	Could we just have "design for use as in therapeutic and diagnostic procedures?" Keep it super broad?
Carl Simon	Then you could add on things on top of it such as "an instructive biomaterial." It would give you some ability to think about "control."
Carl Simon	I was agreeing with Elizabeth and saying that perhaps this is what Bill is getting at, perhaps the biomaterial could be very generic, but you could then think about adding an additional definition on the front such as an instructive material that brings in the idea of control or driving a desired response through an engineered process. But the biomaterial itself doesn't necessarily have to have that specificity.
Serena Best	Can we not just have "designed to interact with living systems?"
David Williams:	I do not think so because it has got to be deliberate, that is why you have controlled, it is a deliberate interaction, not just one that is taking place without any control over it. Or without any intention.
Laura Poole-Warren	What about actually referring to "a material" rather than a substance? So "a material designed for use in a diagnostic and therapeutic application?"
Peter Ma	I also question the very beginning of the definition We said, "has been designed." In some ways if you're doing something that is not "has been used or designed" you're doing something with a material for the first time, is that considered still a biomaterial?
Kai Zhang	That makes sense.
David Williams	I am not quite sure. Obviously, there are several different options coming up here right now.
Kai Zhang	David, you're being bombarded. Let's take them one at a time. Let us take the simplest one. Peter. How would you feel if we said,

"substances designed to take." He's concerned about the past tense. I personally am not concerned. I like it as it is. He's concerned about the use "that has been designed."

Kam Leong	We're doing something new. Has not been designed.
David Williams	Do you mean that anything that's been done before is no longer a biomaterial?
Kam Leong	No.
David Williams	No. I think that is perfect except for the English "that has been designed" that encompasses what you do tomorrow, will have been designed.
Laura Poole-Warren	It is a little bit superfluous though. I think you can remove "has been" it is just a "material designed to" I don't think you need the "has been."
Rena Bizios	In respect to this tense question, the present perfect indicates an action that started in the past and continues in the present, according to grammatic definition. Therefore, this particular definition, "has been" in my opinion encompasses all kinds of materials that have already been designed and formulated and are being used, not only the ones we're preparing today and perhaps in the future. That's why the present will designate a truth and that is another alternative, but I like the present perfect because of the continuity.
Xingdong Zhang	I say the difference between biomaterials and drugs; with this definition, we can understand the difference, between biomaterials and drugs.
David Williams	I think we have taken care of that by talking about substance which "takes a form." A drug is not taking a form. I think that does emphasize the difference between that. We could say "a material." I have no objection to "material" instead of "substance."
Kam Leong	I do think "material" make better sense because we are talking about biomaterials, which are materials.
Kai Zhang	What about bioactive materials? So we get the word in front of "the substance" or the "material."
David Williams	I have changed "substance" to "material." I think that was receiving a fair amount of approval. Okay. How does that sound.
Carl Simon	Yes, that is right. That looks good.
David Williams	Okay. So we move on from that?
Kai Zhang	Are we all okay with this? Then we should move to the next term.
James Anderson	Are we voting on this?
David Williams	I thought we were going through and modifying and then we come back to vote. I am happy if you want to take a vote now.
Carl Simon	I think we should do the vote now.

Kai Zhang	It should be "in the course of any therapeutic;" there are missing words. We are moving forward. Seems like people want to take the vote. On your module it is "one" for yes, "two" for no "three" for abstain. We have the term. We have the vote. Go ahead Carl.

(d) Final Definition and Voting for "Biomaterial"

Biomaterial

A material designed to take a form which can direct, through interactions with living systems, the course of any therapeutic or diagnostic procedure

Voting Yes	41
Voting No	4
Abstain	3
Total Votes	48
Number voting Yes or No	45
Percentage Yes Votes	91.1%

The definition achieved Consensus, having more than 75% Yes votes, with absolute number greater than 30.

(e) Further Commentary on the Definition of "Biomaterial"

Several points arise. First, in the context that David Williams was given the authority to make minor grammatical alterations, a slightly better wording is as follows, and it is this which is confirmed to have consensus:

Biomaterial

A material designed to take a form that can direct, through interactions with living systems, the course of any therapeutic or diagnostic procedure

Second, there was no enthusiasm for generically including references to human and/or veterinary applications in these definitions.

Third, David Williams, in his presentation, pointed out the increasing use of the term "biomaterial" within the context of forestry and agriculture. For example, one University in the United States has a Biomaterials Initiative, defining biomaterials as "any organic materials extracted from ecosystems, green materials that include wood, mushrooms, edible berries, and plant sap in terrestrial ecosystems, and algae in aquatic ecosystems."[2] Obviously, one scientific community cannot prevent another community using terminology that they believe is proprietary to them, but caution has to be taken to avoid confusion. This position was supported by Nicholas Peppas, who noted *"Other societies and other organizations, as you said, agricultural, and other organizations, have basically captured the term "biomaterials" to describe the area that would include their interest and would make them workers*

---

[2] School of Forestry Resources and Environmental Sciences, Michigan Technological University, 2018, www.mtu.edu.

and players in the field. I have a continuous fight with the American Institute of Chemical Engineers staff and members who want to use the word biomaterials to describe corn stalks and other substances to make ethanol. I think this body should express a very strong view about what we feel is biomaterials and I hope that we will ask these organizations, such as the agricultural societies, to use alternative terminology."

B Biomedical Material

In his preconference notes, David Williams indicated that the 1986 Chester conference did discuss the term "biomedical material" which achieved consensus definition as:

An instrument, apparatus, implement, machine, contrivance, in vitro reagent, or other similar or related article, including any component, part or accessory, which is intended for use in the diagnosis of disease or other conditions, or in the cure, mitigation, treatment or prevention of disease in man

The question arose as to whether there was a need to consider this term at all or whether this community considered it to be synonymous with biomaterial. A show of hands indicated that there was no need for further discussion, indicating that these terms were, indeed, synonymous. The conclusions of this conference would therefore indicate that biomaterial was synonymous with biomedical material with the following definition:

Biomaterial, synonymous with Biomedical Material

A material designed to take a form that can direct, through interactions with living systems, the course of any therapeutic or diagnostic procedure

One further point concerning the terms "biomaterial" and "biomedical material" was raised by several delegates in the context of the phrase "biological material." This was not included in the agenda since it is normally considered to be analogous to a "natural material," or a "substance produced by living organisms," etc., without reference to any medical applications. As noted earlier, one comment was made on this matter by Mario Barbosa:

Mario Barbosa   It's about the beginning and the end of the list of definitions. I have difficulties in distinguishing between "biomaterial," "biological material," and "biomedical material." If you use the definition of biomaterial, based on the application, to me biomedical material is more or less synonymous. The other thing I notice is that there's probably another term which we should use, which is "biological material." Of course, wood is a biological material; bone and skin are biological materials, so maybe tomorrow this idea of introducing new terms could be raised again. I believe that the term biological material is needed somewhere.

This view was not supported and was not discussed further.

III

Biomaterial types

Discussed in Session I, Session III, Session V, and Final General Session

Session I Plenary Presentation: *David Williams*
Session I Moderato: *Kai Zhang*
Session I Reporter: *Carl Simon*
Session III Plenary Presentation: *William Wagner*
Session III Moderator: Cato Laurencin
Session III Reporter: Helen Lu
Session V Plenary Presentation: *Nicholas Peppas*
Session V Moderator: *Kazunori Kataoka*
Session V Reporter: *Maria J. Vicent*
Final Session Moderator: *David Williams*
Final Session Reporters: *Carl Simon, Helen Lu, Serena Best*

This section includes terms that delineate subsets of biomaterials based on their essential material science characteristics, and groups of biomaterials defined by specific unique functional or performance characteristics. Those terms that were discussed and voted on are presented first before a summary of those terms that were included in the agenda but not discussed because of a lack of time; the latter are mentioned here in order to provide an indication of the breadth of the vocabulary and the direction of current thinking.

The essential nature of the arguments here was presented by the Session I plenary speaker as follows:

David Williams   We then come to look at the terms bioceramic, biopolymer, and so on. Let me emphasize that when we look at classes of materials, not just biomaterials but materials themselves, those classes are based upon atomic structure and we see the main groups of metals, polymers, ceramics, together with their derivatives, the composites. There is a temptation in the biomedical field to use directly analogous terms, i.e., biometals, biopolymers, bioceramics and, perhaps, biocomposites. That, however, leads to confusion. There's no consistency in the way which we have used these terms over the last thirty or forty years. It is sensible to look at common usage. The prefix "bio" could refer to "living" or "medical

Definitions of Biomaterials for the Twenty-First Century
DOI: https://doi.org/10.1016/B978-0-12-818291-8.00003-1

application" and this common usage has led to the former meaning in the case of polymers and the latter in the case of ceramics, with little interest in either "biometals" or "biocomposites."

A Bioceramic

(a) Possible Definitions of "Bioceramic" Included in Final Program

Any ceramic, glass or glass-ceramic that is used as a biomaterial

(b) David Williams; Perspectives on "Bioceramic" and Suggested Definition

Let us start with the simplest of these, which is bioceramic. I know a few people have tried to claim that hydroxyapatite is a bioceramic, because it is contained within bones or teeth. I don't think that helps us. My suggestion to you is a bioceramic is "any ceramic, glass or glass-ceramic that is used as a biomaterial." That's clear, unequivocal, but that is up to you to discuss and decide.

(c) Edited Discussion of "Bioceramic"

Iulian Antoniac	I appreciate the definition very much but in order to be more consistent regarding different biomaterial classes, I would like to propose new terms like "ceramic biomaterials" that is not present. Also "biocomposites" could be added to these definitions.
David Williams	Iulian, that's a good point. You've given three possibilities there. I think you're suggesting ceramic biomaterial as well as bioceramic. It's quite possibly under the definition of bioceramic, we could put in brackets, synonymous with ceramic biomaterial. Would that satisfy you?
Changsheng Liu	Bioceramic. Can we include cement, ceramic cement and glass and glass ceramic?
David Williams	Thanks. I think that you can have a cement which is a ceramic. I do not think we need to define what a cement is, bearing in mind that bone cement is a polymeric cement.
Changsheng Liu	Organic cement.
David Williams	As far as material classification is concerned, most cements are ceramics, or maybe glass ceramics, or mixtures. I don't think there is any real difference there. I think it would be hard to separate out a cement in that definition. If you have an inorganic cement it is included, if you have an organic cement it is not.
Changsheng Liu	Cements from the point of view of material science including glass, ceramic and cement. But inorganic material cements belong to the ceramic.
David Williams	I understand that, but we're talking about a "bioceramic" and not all ceramics. I personally think that within the group of terms we normally include as the ceramic group, "ceramic, glass and glass

ceramic" is sufficiently encompassing. If we include the word "cement," we have to say, "but not acrylic cement" or something similar, which does not make a good definition.

Arthur Coury — I consider carbon and its forms as a ceramic. If we do not include it here, do we do it somewhere else?

David Williams — Good point, Art. When I look at the classification of materials, I would have carbon materials as separate class. I would consider metallic systems, polymeric systems. ceramic systems, carbon systems and then composites. I do not include carbons with ceramics here. At one time, but to a much lesser extent today, we had vitreous carbon, yes that was ceramic as it glass-like, but now I am not sure I would want to put graphene and fullerenes in with ceramics. In view of time constraints, I did not include carbon-based biomaterials in the agenda.

Kai Zhang — David, is necessary to include glass in bioceramics?

David Williams — Yes. I think so. There are quite a few glasses and glass ceramics used in orthopedics.

Kai Zhang — Then the bioceramics will include bioglass?

David Williams — Yes. Serena you'd agree with that?

Serena Best — Yes.

Xingdong Zhang — I think, David, the glass or glass ceramic, I think the ceramic matrix composite maybe belongs to the ceramics.

David Williams — Sorry, which composite?

Xingdong Zhang — Ceramic matrix.

David Williams — A ceramic matrix?

Xingdong Zhang — Yes.

David Williams — What is the other phase in the composite?

Changsheng Liu — On that point, if it includes the cement, and include glass, but glass is non-crystalline, so the ceramic sometimes crack and maybe a glass or ceramic. In the point of view of materials science, the ceramic, the three kinds of ceramic, glass and cement. So, normally they are a crystal structure.

David Williams — If I have understood you, there are amorphous ceramics used as biomaterials. There are amorphous glass phosphates, for example.

Peter Ma — Overall I agree with this definition. I understand that there is a difference from materials science. The ceramic is different from glass. Ceramics may have a crystal structure, but glass does not. But phosphates have both crystalline and amorphous components.

David Williams — Yes.

Peter Ma — But if we define it this way, I am fine with that. We just have to include any inorganic material, right? Both glass or ceramic in this concept.

| Arthur Coury | Sorry, before voting, David you mentioned that it is synonymous with "ceramic biomaterials." |
| Carl Simon | I was just going to say, he already handled it. I think you have mine. |

(d) Final Definition and Voting for "Bioceramic"

Bioceramic, synonymous with Ceramic Biomaterial

Any ceramic, glass or glass-ceramic that is used as a biomaterial

Voting Yes	40
Voting No	4
Abstain	4
Total Votes	48
Number voting Yes or No	44
Percentage Yes Votes	90.9%

The definition achieved Consensus, having more than 75% Yes votes, with absolute number greater than 30.

B Biopolymer

(a) Possible Definitions of "Biopolymer" Included in Final Program

1. Naturally occurring long-chain molecules
2. A polymeric substance formed in a biological system
3. A polymer synthesized by a living organism

(b) David Williams; Perspectives on "Biopolymer" and Suggested Definition

Let me now come to "biopolymer"; the same is not true here as it was for a "bioceramic." "Biopolymer," in fact, is rarely used to refer to medical applications. Instead a biopolymer is usually considered to be one of the following: (1) naturally occurring long-chain molecules, (2) a polymeric substance formed in a biological system, or (3) a polymer synthesized by living organisms. I do not have a tremendous preference there, but with a slight leaning towards the latter. This really comes into focus when we consider polymeric materials used in tissue engineering applications where we see a very clear distinction now between synthetic polymers and natural biopolymers. I think option three is preferred.

It follows that we may wish to look at that alternative to "bioceramic" and I think most people would say "a polymeric biomaterial," which I believe is synonymous with "a biomedical polymer," and that may be defined as "any polymeric material, either natural or synthetic, used as a biomaterial."

(c) Edited Discussion of "Biopolymer"

Kristi Anseth	I want to come back to the point of biopolymers and that definition. I am an editor for *Biomacromolecules*. I think some of the confusion, especially with polymers, is whether you're talking about single chains, single molecules, versus assembling those chains into a material and its associated structure. I was curious if your biopolymer definition might be tightened up some. Are we talking about proteins? But, yet, how one might … So, you have collagen as a protein, but then how you would assemble it and make it into a matrix, then maybe the collagen matrix is a biomaterial. The biopolymer, the biomacromolecule would be the single protein.
David Williams	I understand that the problem if you're tightening this definition, as you say, then you may get too specific. For example, I think biopolymers include polysaccharides as well as collagens. I would like it to be as broad as possible.
Kristi Anseth	Right, yes. A polysaccharide, though, can be a single polymer chain. I am just saying, maybe it's something we should think about, with scale, because we come to the same thing with nanostructures, because materials do not have to do anything in bulk, and with polymers, I think, especially it becomes very different. Are you talking about this heterogeneous collection of chains that make a material, or are you talking about single molecules?
David Williams	I totally accept what you say. A basic principle I have had here is that our definition should be self-contained and then we may want to amplify that when putting it into context. I have been rather careful not to include too much detail, which is highly specific, or indeed gives mechanisms. Again, that's just my view.
Carl Simon	Kristi, you had brought up the issue of biomacromolecules? Do you want to pursue this?
Kristi Anseth	So you could change it to be "macromolecules synthesized by living organisms" if you don't want to use polymer in the definition.
David Williams	I am happy with that. Does everybody agree to change that to "macromolecule."
Arthur Coury:	Yes.
Elizabeth Cosgriff-H	Yes.
John Ramshaw	David, does it include polymers made just by enzymatic synthesis?
Carl Simon	Are all macromolecules polymers? Because if they're not then we shouldn't make that change, because it is "biopolymer" that we are talking about.

John Ramshaw	David, if somebody makes a polymer by enzymatic synthesis is that covered or not?
Carl Simon	Nicholas, are all macromolecules polymers?
Nicholas Peppas	I think so. They are, but I have another question. So are you telling me that I can never call in my papers polyvinyl alcohol a biopolymer. That's what you're telling me right now. I cannot. Because it's not made by a living organism?
Carl Simon	If you're following these definitions, then yes.
Nicholas Peppas	I cannot vote for that. I do not know what to suggest, but I cannot vote for that.
David Williams	I suggest we vote on number three and if we do not achieve consensus we can come back, otherwise we'll be here all day.
Peter Ma	Yes. I would rather change back to "polymer" rather than "macromolecule" because I think the terms "polymer" and "biopolymer" are the terms that we are trying to define. I would rather have the word "polymer" than "macromolecule" in the definition.
David Williams	I don't normally like doing this, but could we say "a macromolecule or polymer."
Peter Ma	Yes, I guess so. I would go with that.
David Williams	Fair enough. Cato what do you prefer? Macromolecule or polymer.
Cato Laurencin	I think "polymer" because some substances may be macromolecules, but they're not polymers.
Carl Simon	Is there a difference between macromolecule and polymer? Or are they the same thing?
Kristi Anseth	Yes.
Carl Simon	David, you want to change it back to polymer? It sounds like the mood has swung.
David Williams	I'm seeing equal numbers.
Carl Simon	We could take a vote and if it doesn't pass we could change it to polymer and take another quick vote.
David Williams	Why don't we have a quick show of hands? Informal show of hands for polymer or macromolecule. Then we vote on three. So all those who would favor polymer. All those who favor macromolecule. I go back to polymer. Sorry Kristi.
Joachim Kohn	Why do you do this? A macromolecule is just a large molecule. A polymer consists of repeat units that are repeating themselves; monomers. They are chained together. They are not the same and polymer is what we actually want here.
David Williams	Fine, I agree.
Kristi Anseth	Okay, but then a protein does not count here. A protein would not count here.

(d) Final Definition and Voting for Biopolymer

The wording of definition (3) was changed back to "A polymer synthesized by living organisms," although there continued to be separate conversations in the room about this. The general feeling was that "polymer" was more relevant than "macromolecule" and it was subsequently noted that there is still scientific discussion in the literature about whether proteins are polymers. The consensus was that proteins are biopolymers, reinforced by the commentary in a recent publication on biomedical biopolymers to the effect that the US Congress Office of Technology Assessment classifies biopolymers into nucleic acids, proteins, polysaccharides, polyhydroxyalkanoates and polyphenols.[1]

The definitive view of the delegates was summed up as follows:

Arthur Coury So, may I please make a comment. I am a polymer scientist and I have always stated that a polymer is a large molecule made up of repeating units of smaller molecules. And a protein is a polypeptide. It is made up of units of amino acids. To me, it is a polymer, even though it might have one molecule away, it is still a polymer. I think you could probably have a large molecule that is not polymeric. And so, I think they are distinct, and we should refer to polymers.

Voting on this rather contentious issue was therefore based on the following term:

Biopolymer

A polymer synthesized by living organisms

Voting Yes	37
Voting No	12
Abstain	1
Total Votes	50
Number voting Yes or No	49
Percentage Yes Votes	75.5%

The definition achieved Consensus, having more than 75% Yes votes, with absolute number greater than 30.

The vote was clearly marginal, the division largely being based on the polymer versus macromolecule issue. The Executive Committee had, during its preconference deliberations, decided that in some circumstances more than one definition could be discussed, and voted on. This was based on situations where identical terms had been developed within their own disciplines and could then be juxtaposed within multidisciplinary areas such as biomedical engineering, very correctly but possibly confusingly; examples include dislocation (in crystallographic defects and musculoskeletal trauma), and fatigue (in mechanical properties of materials and internal medicine). Several delegates thought that

---

[1] Yaday P, et al., Biomedical biopolymers, their origin and evolution in biomedical sciences: A systematic review, J Clin Diagn Res, 2015;9(9):Ze21-25.

all three proposed definitions, which were quite similar and were all essentially correct scientifically, should be voted for inclusion. This was done, and the voting to include all three was as follows:

Voting Yes	32
Voting No	17
Abstain	1
Total Votes	50
Number voting Yes or No	49
Percentage Yes Votes	65.3%

This did qualify for provisional consensus, but this became a moot point since the preferred definition did achieve consensus, confirmed as follows:

Biopolymer

A polymer synthesized by living organisms

(e) Comments on Polymeric Biomaterial and Metallic Biomaterial

The Conference Program showed that the following two terms were scheduled for discussion in Session I, with proposed definitions:

Polymeric Biomaterial (**synonymous with** *Biomedical Polymer*)
Any polymeric material, either natural or synthetic, that is used as a biomaterial
Metallic Biomaterial
Any metallic material that is used as a biomaterial

In the introductory comments for the session, the following points were made:

David Williams	It follows that we may wish to look at that some terms are similar to bioceramic; I think most people would agree that a polymeric biomaterial, which I believe is synonymous with a biomedical polymer, may be defined as "any polymeric material, either natural or synthetic used as a biomaterial."
David Williams	The difficult one is "biometal." There is a journal called *Biometals.* Occasionally biometal is used to describe a metallic element that has biochemical function. It is very difficult to define those; for example zinc, iron and others are incorporated into tissue as essential trace elements, but that to me is not a very good definition or concept of biometal. I do not think the term "biometal" has any use in biomedical materials or biomaterials contexts. So I prefer "metallic biomaterial," which should be defined as "any metallic material used as a biomaterial." That's something people might argue, are we talking about pure metals or alloys which are very different. I do not think we should distinguish these. Metals and alloys, they're all metallic materials.

There was no time to discuss either of these definitions, but it is logical to conclude, because of the analogous use of the now-accepted term "bioceramic," these two would likely have achieved consensus should they have been discussed.

C Hydrogel

(a) Possible Definitions of "Hydrogel" Included in Final Program

1. A physically or chemically crosslinked polymer swollen in water (or biological fluids)
2. A three-dimensional, water-swollen structure composed of hydrophilic homopolymers or co-polymers

(b) Nicholas Peppas; Perspectives on "Hydrogel" and Suggested Definition

Nicholas Peppas   It has been suggested that the word hydrogel be defined here because hydrogels are very important materials in the drug delivery field, but they are also important materials elsewhere in our biomaterials field. So I have come almost verbatim with the same definition that I gave about 32 years ago; "physically or chemically cross-linked polymer swollen in water" and I have added "or biological fluids" since we are in the biomedical field. Let me explain a little bit more about the terms "physically" and "chemically." Of course, chemical crosslinking is the main characteristic of hydrogels, especially covalent bonding, but as you can imagine you can have ionic bonding, you can have complexation. You can have simply chain entanglements that are permanent junctions. Thus keeping the word "physically" here adds that component. In the definition, if it is just chemically cross-linked, I believe it has to be swollen in water.

Nicholas Peppas   Swollen in water, I hope the word swelling is understood, and I used the term "biological fluids"; you could use "physiological fluids" if you prefer. Or it could be a physiological fluid or a biological fluid.

Nicholas Peppas   The second option/definition is a slight different version. It was proposed by one of my colleagues. It talks about having a hydrophilic copolymer, the purpose of which is to swell the material. So hydrogel is different than a cross-link network because it does have to have water. We do not specify what percentage of water is needed; we leave it undefined. If 5% water is enough to be called hydrogels or 90% water, we don't care right now.

(c) Edited Discussion of "Hydrogel"

Carl Simon   Do you think the word "network" should be after "polymer" giving "polymer network" because I always think of a network.

Nicholas Peppas	Network is a cross-linked polymer, so we can't say cross-linked network as it gives a double intention. It has to be a network or a cross-linked polymer. If we say a network I am afraid some people who are not in the field will be confused. So is it a polymer or not? That is why I am staying with cross-linked polymer.
Arthur Coury	I have been working with hydrogels for decades. I have grappled with this and when I teach it I always say at the time of delivery because you say 20% water, you have an electrode with 20% water that you deliver at the time as a solid hydrogel. It has to be self-supporting, I think, but sometimes that is really not cross-linked in the ultimate sense that if it takes on more water it is going to dissolve, so I always, in my teaching, say "at the time of delivery."
Nicholas Peppas	No I understand what you mean and that's a very well taken point, but here the term, at least as we are presenting it to you, is a more general term which will help us also in other biomaterials areas, not only in drug delivery.
Kristi Anseth	I really like the first one and I think it captures almost all the ways I would use hydrogels to describe new material systems.
John Ramshaw	Could you clarify, please, in relation to the second definition, are you seeing a hydrogel as having a distinct shape and form and so would you therefore include injectable hydrogels, or not. I am also happy that I think it is a commonly used polymer. The original hydrogels were not polymer materials at all. I think that's archaic and can be forgotten.
Nicholas Peppas	The first term includes the so-called hydrocolloids as the systems that were first available, 50, 70 years ago. The pectin, agar and so on. They are gels. Are they hydrogels? They do incorporate water, but they do dissolve very easily as Art said.
Nicholas Peppas	Ah you were thinking of…, That is… the three-dimensional material obviously is not going to be injectable. It cannot be injected. I think the second term is not really a very well-defined term. I think we should stay with the first one.
John Ramshaw	So yours would not have a specific shape or form.
Nicholas Peppas	Yes. Not specific.
Guoping Chen	For the definition, can we change the "or" to "and/or"? Because hydrogels can be physical and chemical; not only physical or chemical.
Nicholas Peppas	The term "and/or" here will give the impression that there have to be both chemical and physical cross-links. I agree with you that in many systems of high molecular weight when they are cross-linked, some cross-links are followed by entanglements and others are formed by covalent bonding, but the general idea is that whether we refer to physical cross-links or chemical cross-links we incorporate them in this definition. They are included in the term.

James Anderson	My question is for the first one. Why include water? It is a biological fluid that we are really interested in.
Nicholas Peppas	You are absolutely right.
James Anderson	I would delete water.
Nicholas Peppas	You are absolutely right. I included water because most people in the laboratory when they start-
James Anderson	Yes but what we are talking about is the delivery into a patient, we're not talking about what sits on the bench top.
Guoping Chen	Okay.
James Anderson	Or perhaps I have that wrong.
David Williams	I think substantially right, Jim, but bear in mind we use hydrogels *ex vivo* in tissue engineering applications and they're not directly in the patient at that point.
James Anderson	But still in contact with biological fluids.
David Williams	Putting it into context.
Kai Zhang	I like the first definition. I am just trying to see in the water and then in parenthesis of biological fluids. Can we do something about aqueous medium. I don't know what you really mean by biological fluids — blood maybe?
Nicholas Peppas	The term water is there because traditionally since the days of Flory, gel and hydrogel are defined in water, not in biological fluids. In a biological fluid, that same gel is going to be slightly shrunk because of the ionic strength.
Nicholas Peppas	Now we say biological fluids because here we're talking about drug delivery. In other applications of biomaterials, we are talking about contact with physiological fluids. I want to make sure that's incorporated. It could be peptides, it could be proteins, it could be enzymes in solutions so yes aqueous media would be a good definition. Typically, I try to avoid difficult Latin terms in definitions because not everybody knows Latin as well. They'll say what is this aqueous medium. We can do whatever you want.
Arthur Coury	I feel obliged to mention that in our field it is always going to be a polymer, but there are self-supporting gels that are formed with silica, for example, at certain concentrations, and when you dry them down you call them xerogels. There is some of that in our field, but I don't know if we should have a statement about this because there are certainly other hydrogels that are not polymer based.
Andrés García	I agree with Kristi. The first definition is accurate, and I suggest we vote and approve on that.
Nicholas Peppas	Let me make one small change. I have removed the second definition. If you want me remove the parentheses or biological fluids or just leave it all biological fluids, but without the parentheses.

Rena Bizios	Without parentheses.
Nicholas Peppas	Without parentheses. Let's look at this and tell me how you feel about that.
Kazunori Kataoka	Okay. Any comments? Or just on this?
John Brash	I hesitate to go to back to try to differentiate between polymer and polymeric material. We discussed that quite well yesterday, I believe, but in my mind polymer conjures up the idea of a single polymer molecule, which is not the idea here, so I would prefer to see polymeric material as opposed to polymer.
David Williams	I agree with that.
Nicholas Peppas	I would like to see it staying as polymer. I am coming from polymer science, of course, when I make a point. It is a network structure, molecular, that absorbs water. Is it also a material? Of course, it is a material at the same time, but I think we try to define the hydrogel itself here.
Kristi Anseth	I think we do not talk about metal materials, ceramic materials. So, polymer is descriptive. Usually, if we want to differentiate, we would call a polymer chain. I advocate for polymer.
Kazunori Kataoka	In terms of polymer science, we think about strings or micromolecules. But in the case of the polymer, it's more like a network or products or materials.
Joachim Kohn	I am sorry if I misunderstood. I also would like to endorse that we stay with polymer. I support Kristi.
John Ramshaw	Are you including gelatin in your grouping of polymers?
Nicholas Peppas	Yes, it is a major form of denatured collagen.
Kazunori Kataoka	Yes.
Kazunori Kataoka	Okay, so if there are no further comments, we direct to wrap up the discussion, and maybe move into vote.

(d) Final Definition and Voting for "Hydrogel"

Hydrogel

A physically or chemically cross-linked polymer, swollen in water or biological fluids

Voting Yes	42
Voting No	2
Abstain	0
Total Votes	44
Number voting Yes or No	44
Percentage Yes Votes	95.4%

The definition achieved Consensus, having more than 75% Yes votes, with absolute number greater than 30.

D BioHybrid Material

(a) Possible Definitions of "Biohybrid Material" Included in Final Program

A biomaterial that is comprised of materials derived from both natural and synthetic sources

(b) William Wagner; Perspectives on "Biohybrid Material" and Suggested Definition

William Wagner	This is pretty simple, but perhaps controversial, I don't know. Again, it's a term that appears quite a bit in the literature, including the biomaterials literature. This seems, to me, to be about the simplest way to describe what most people mean when they say biohybrid. The suggested definition is, therefore "A biomaterial that is comprised of materials derived from both natural and synthetic sources."

(c) Edited Discussion of "Biohybrid Material"

Deon Bezuidenhout	How does that differ from a "hybrid biomaterial"? Biohybrid implies to me something that … There might be some hybridization in the "bio" aspect. Is that just how it's used most often? Or, how would that differ from a hybrid biomaterial?
William Wagner	I don't know how it would. I would consider those to be synonymous. Except for the fact that, what I see is more people using the term biohybrid in literature, than hybrid biomaterial.
Carl Simon	It seems like it ought to be hybrid biomaterial. I agree with Deon. If it is biohybrid material, then maybe the definition should include a material that "is comprised of," not a biomaterial.
William Wagner	The reason it says a biomaterial is because these are used in this context, as a biomaterial that has already been defined, so not something that would be used in industry for some other application.
Rena Bizios	Let me rephrase that, please. I'm sorry. Does Bill answer your question? Because I understood it differently. You're not questioning "biomaterial." You are questioning the "biohybrid." If you put "hybrid biomaterial," it is fine according to Carl, right?
Carl Simon	Yes. As it is, I would probably vote no, because it is just another term we don't really need, and if people are using it, maybe they should not be. Maybe we should not endorse this word.
Nicholas Peppas	Yes, I hear with significant interest Carl's comment, and he comes from the right place, but most of us use the term biohybrid, and I

do not want to shake the waters too much today; I will stay with "biohybrid." However, I am not very confident with the end of the definition. It's comprised of synthetic and natural components, or synthetic and natural materials. I would prefer synthetic and natural components, because if it is an antibody attached to a synthetic polymer, it is a biohybrid. That's why I say components. That covers a large range of systems. As for the biohybrid, Carl, I agree with you, it should be called hybrid biomaterial, but the thing is, change everything right now?

William Wagner
This is one of the issues, I think, with the dictionary, too. If one were to lay out the English language, we certainly would not have the mess that we have right now with it, but the dictionary seeks to capture words that are commonly used, and I think part of that is what we want to do. Although, in some cases, and I think biomaterial, again, is a great example. We're trying to draw a line in the sand and say, "No, we claim this term for this type of definition."

Iulian Antoniac
Maybe a good solution to what is synonymous to hybrid biomaterials, because there are also hybrid materials, and also, it is confirmed that people could understand that would be a combination but biological sources, when we will add just biohybrid materials.

David Williams
I think I understood what Carl was saying, but the same argument could be put from the other end of hybrid biomaterial. I thought I was going to agree with Deon, but then, when you think about it, a hybrid biomaterial does not imply any biological, or natural, source. It could be two totally different synthetic ones. I do not like either. If I had to do one, I prefer biohybrid.

John Brash
Yes, just for the record, I like a hybrid biomaterial rather than biohybrid material. I'm not going to give any argument, but as an editorial point, the English should not be "comprised of," it should be "comprises," or, "is composed of."

Nicholas Peppas
The only thing I wanted to add is, I do not have access to Google of course, here, but I do have access to Baidu, and the word biohybrid material appears quite a lot. For example, one journal gives "A biohybrid consists of a living organism, or cell, and at least one engineered component." That recurring theme appears in several other definitions, in good journals. RSC journals and so forth.

Cato Laurencin
All right, we have got a healthy debate. Want to vote and see where we are in terms of that?

Rena Bizios
One thing, I like what Nicholas had suggested, to make it composed of both natural and synthetic components, and take out

	the, "derived from." It's not only derivation, it is a combination. Bringing together those things. Composed of, yes. But derived is becomes now, composed from . . . of both natural and synthetic components.
Arthur Coury	I hope if nothing goes up on the board that at least my comments are being recorded. I am not so sure about that, but in the next section, we are going to speak about hybrid organs, and we call them hybrid bioartificial organs, and we hope that that term gets taken up, because I think that fully explains and is accurate. You might say hybrid bioartificial material.
Mário Barbosa	I wonder whether natural could be replaced by biological, because a rock is natural, but not biological.
William Wagner	Let's get the vote.
Cato Laurencin	All right. Are we ready to vote?
Cato Laurencin	Is everyone happy? Okay, let us vote now. One for yes for this. Two for no.

(d) Final Definition and Voting for "Biohybrid Material"

Biohybrid Material

A biomaterial that is composed of both biological and synthetic components

Voting Yes	36
Voting No	13
Abstain	0
Total Votes	49
Number voting Yes or No	49
Percentage Yes Votes	73.5%

The definition did not achieve Consensus, having less than 75% Yes votes. With 73.5% Yes votes and an absolute number of 36 votes, it did achieve provisional consensus.

(e) Further Commentary on the Definition of "Biohybrid Material"

The preferred definition did not achieve consensus largely because of different views on whether we should be discussing biohybrid material or hybrid biomaterial. Examination of multiple dictionaries after the conference suggest that the correct interpretation has been used here, "biohybrid" generally being considered to mean "containing or composed of both biological and non-biological components." Furthermore, when used as an adjective, 'hybrid' means something composed of two different types of component, without any implication that at least one of them has a biological nature; this is important in the context of the structure and application of biomaterials. This does not really address the sensible comment of Arthur Coury with reference to hybrid bioartificial organs, but the conference did not have time to discuss that.

E Responsive Biomaterial (considered along with smart material and intelligent material)

Editor's Note: The three adjectives "smart," "intelligent," and "responsive" were all scheduled for consideration in Session V. Some suggested definitions were included in the conference papers. The discussions, not surprisingly proved contentious. As the following text shows, consensus was reached for "responsive biomaterial." The use of "smart material" in the biomedical context was largely disapproved, while there was general agreement that the concept of "intelligent materials" was valid but rather difficult to incorporate into a definition.

(a) Possible Definitions of "Intelligent and Responsive Materials" Included in Final Program

Intelligent biomaterial
A biomaterial that responds to its environment in response to pH- or temperature changes

Environmentally responsive biomaterial
A biomaterial that exhibit swelling behavior dependent on the external environment

(b) Nicholas Peppas; Perspectives on "Smart, Intelligent and Responsive Materials" and Suggested Definition

Nicholas Peppas	And now for "intelligent material." It was suggested yesterday and discussed that we add the word "smart." You decide whether you want to keep just "smart," just "intelligent," or both. Of various explanations, definitions, we decided to go with the definition in Ratner's Book[2] of "whose physical stage is altered in response to pH, temperature, ionic strength, or other environmental inputs or input." We have slightly modified this but that is the definition we are proposing.
Nicholas Peppas	Since I say, "see also next definition," I wanted to show you the next definition, "environmentally responsible material." Some people like to use that word. "The biomaterial that exhibits swelling, shrinking or other physical modification behavior dependent on the external environment." If we go back to the first one, the idea all of you recognize is that you have a thermodynamic system which responds to the surrounding fluid. This is very important for drug delivery. The pH change will lead to drug release. The temperature change, as Okano, Hoffman, and many others have told us, would lead to drug release, and of course Kataoka, ionic strength will lead to drug release, and so on. So that is really the intent.

[2] Ratner B, et al, Biomaterials Science; An Introduction to Materials in Medicine, Academic Press, 3rd edition, 2012.

(c) Edited Discussion of "Smart, Intelligent and Responsive Materials"

Hua Ai	Okay, it is good, first, but we have to change the way to say it. Some materials were not designed to change with pH or temperature or ionic strengths, just because of the design. But I think this should be intentionally designed for this response. Some of these materials, because the side effects, are not designed to respond to pH. So I think maybe we should not use, it is altered, maybe it is designed in response, or some other phrase.
Nicholas Peppas	You are proposing a biomaterial whose physical state is designed in response?
Laura Poole-Warren	I was actually just going to make a very similar point. I think the factor of intent is not actually in there, so I think we do need to include some form of the intent. So, "designed to have a predicted response in," I guess, in response to factors in the internal or external environment. Something like that. I think going into pH, temperature, ionic strength, or other environmental input is too much detail. I think you can just say, "in response to the internal or external environment." "Designed to have a predictable response to factors in the internal and/or external environment, or just the environment," I guess.
Joachim Kohn	Nicholas, please allow me to make a more provocative statement. I think that there are certain terms that have crept into science that don't belong there. For instance, many people speak about happy cells, instead of saying they are viable or something. It's just bad use of the word. I know that smart biomaterials is used very commonly, but if you really think about it, it is a bad term. It is a slang term that means almost nothing. And I think that this body has an opportunity perhaps to discourage the continuous use of this slang in science.
Joachim Kohn	My suggestion would be to not endorse the word "smart" in the definition, and perhaps even to go one step further, and that's the controversial part. Perhaps you can include in the document at one point that the term "smart biomaterials" is actually slang and should not be used. That would be entirely optional. The definition itself is very good, but that smart is something that, Nicholas, you may want to consider.
Nicholas Peppas	So, you are against the word "smart"?
Joachim Kohn	Yes, I am.
Nicholas Peppas	And in favor of the word "intelligent," or you don't want that either?
Joachim Kohn	Smart is ... you know we have a smart car. Smart is really slang. "Intelligent" could be fine, because intelligent speaks about intelligent design or something. I can see that better. I am not against the definition in any way. I just wanted to make that point.

David Williams	I absolutely, totally agree, I have never liked the terms either "smart" or "intelligent," because those imply intrinsic ability to change something. We are talking about responsive materials. In other words, they are responding, whether it's the environment or some stimulus. I would like to delete, permanently delete, both "smart" and "intelligent," and just talk about "responsive" biomaterials.
Joachim Kohn	But, because it's so widely used, you're going to have to have a statement that you have discouraged the use of these words, and that makes an impact perhaps on the field.
David Williams	I absolutely agree.
Jiandong Ding	One term could have added significantly, because if we change temperature, any material will be changed more or less. But for intelligent material, it means have a "significant" change. So I think maybe added this term. For instance, "the physical state is significantly altered in response to . . ."
Nicholas Peppas	I would like to make a few comments about this. We have a thermodynamic system that consists of various components. The system is not an ideal thermodynamic system. Nothing works like ideal gases. Typically, you have a real thermodynamic system with activity coefficients significantly different than one.
Nicholas Peppas	When we started in the biomaterials field, many of our forefathers, naively, they were talking about polymers, and they were adding the polymers in saline, and they thought that that was the solution of the problem. Well, it is not. A polymeric material that is cross-linked, that has hydroxyl groups, that has amino groups, that has other groups on it, responds to the surrounding environment. This is a thermodynamic interaction. It's a real thermodynamic interaction. The system is not ideal. It is real and it responds to the surrounding environment.
Nicholas Peppas	I am willing to accept the word "responsive" that David and Joachim suggested. But I cannot give up the word "intelligent." The material has the ability to recognize the surrounding system. When I create a new material, when Laura Kiessling at Wisconsin creates a new material that recognizes glucose, it recognizes glucose over galactose. It has the ability to capture just glucose, not galactose. That is an intelligent system.
Nicholas Peppas	I do not like the word "smart." It was suggested by others. I think it is a slang term. I do not want to have it. But I cannot really say that people who work on intelligent materials do not understand what they are doing. They understand thermodynamics much better than any of us.
Nicholas Peppas	So, I will go with what you want here, but in the Chengdu Manifesto, I am not going to sign a document that says there is no

	such a thing as an "intelligent biomaterial." I disagree with that part. I am willing to say here, let's call it . . . That's why I presented a second term. Let's take again the term "responsive biomaterial" and put it here in the first.
Kazunori Kataoka	That is an alternative?
James Anderson	Yes, I wanted to come back to an earlier comment that Laura had made. I think that the terms "design" and "prediction" should be included in this definition.
Nicholas Peppas	Okay, I am willing to . . .
James Anderson	Biomaterial whose physical state is designed to be altered in response . . . How did you say it?
Nicholas Peppas	Is designed to have a predictable response
Nicholas Peppas	To factors. Laura, did you say "to factors?"
Laura Poole-Warren	Yes. To factors in the environment or the internal and external environments.
Nicholas Peppas	Environment.
James Anderson	Yes, I think the terms design and prediction put this on a much firmer scientific ground than the terms, "intelligent" and "smart." If I use those definitions, I can assume that any physical chemical change is intelligent or smart, and in fact, it is not. You know that.
Nicholas Peppas	Let me try to modify what you said.
Xiaobing Fu	My definition is smart biomaterials, they have ability to regulate the pH, temperature. Not a posteriori. It is supposed to regulate the condition. So, your definition is not a posteriori. It is the material that is suitable to the condition. Smart materials should have the ability to regulate their conditions based on their physical condition, their dissolution, their ability. So these are smart, intelligent biomaterials. It is my opinion.
Kazunori Kataoka	Okay. So that means it may be similar to design or, design or predictor. Is that correct? Is that what you mean? What do you say about order?
John Ramshaw	I would like to agree with David on "responsive." I do not like the word "smart." Never have done. Always assumed it was something people put in grants to make them sound trendy, and prefer to be left to the realm of the tabloid press.
Nicholas Peppas	Laura, David, Jim, or anybody who suggested. Please look at this definition which includes your comments, your terms.
Laura Poole-Warren	Not "by factoring in," but "by factors."
James Anderson	It is the response to external environmental conditions.
Nicholas Peppas	To have a predictable response to environmental conditions.
Kazunori Kataoka	To have a predictable response.

Maria J. Vicent	They asked him to delete the word "external."
Nicholas Peppas	Do you want me to delete the word "external"?
David Williams	I think that's fine. I'm happy with that, Nick. I think we have agreed to eliminate the word "smart." I am understanding that several people like the word "intelligent" for a variety of reasons, and we have to recognize that it is there. I suggest that we vote on that definition, but there will be something in the text, some note to recognize the importance of intelligence. Perhaps Nick, you and I could discuss exactly what that note should be, as a caveat to that.
Nicholas Peppas	I am comfortable with this, if that's what you want. That does not mean that I bury the word "intelligent."
David Williams	That is what I am saying. Rather than bury the word intelligent, I am saying, let us as recognize that all of the materials we are talking about are responsive, but let us add a caveat to that as a note saying, this should take into account the context of intelligence.
Nicholas Peppas	Okay.

(d) Final Definition and Voting for "Responsive Biomaterial"

Responsive Biomaterial

A biomaterial whose physical state is designed to have a predictable response to external environmental conditions

Voting Yes	44
Voting No	1
Abstain	2
Total Votes	47
Number voting Yes or No	45
Percentage Yes Votes	97.8%

The definition achieved Consensus, having more than 75% Yes votes, with absolute number greater than 30.

F Tissue Inducing Biomaterial

(a) Possible Definitions of "Tissue Inducing Biomaterial" Included in Final Program

No preliminary definitions were provided since the term was not in the original agenda

(b) Xingdong Zhang and Kai Zhang; Perspectives on "Tissue-Inducing Biomaterials" and Suggested Definition

Kai Zhang	On behalf of Professor Xingdong Zhang, we have this concept, called tissue inducing biomaterials, read as following "Appropriately designed material that could regenerate damaged tissues or organs, without addition of any living cells and/or growth factors."
Kai Zhang	This definition is based on the finding of Professor Zhang, first identified in 1991, with the biphasic calcium phosphate, that the material self-developed ectopic bone formation in animal models. And in 1993, Klaus DeGroot from the Netherlands also demonstrated the same concept with bioactive ceramics. And then Professor Kokubo from Japan, through the 90s and also mainly in early 2000s, showed that the porous titanium with bioactive surfaces conducted similar ectopic bone formation.
Kai Zhang	And later, Professor Xingdong Zhang's group at Sichuan University has been doing a lot of research for different tissues other than bone, but also cartilage, and recently tendon and ligament. So the material, the original material, biphasic calcium phosphate material has been commercialized in China as a bone void filler, and has been sold hundreds and thousands of units. He himself and his group has got a lot of credit for this finding, and also the translation to the clinical application.
David Williams	Thank you Kai. Professor Zhang, you want to add to that, please?
Xingdong Zhang	We have finally found that materials can induce cartilage to regenerate, and it has passed the animal experiments, and is in clinical trial now. Some people also found their materials can induce ligaments to regenerate, and is also in the clinical testing. I think this is an important direction, so we have to give the definition. This is my suggestion, yes.

(c) Edited Discussion of "Tissue Inducing Biomaterials"

Jiandong Ding	I think this is a very important concept and term. But I would like to make some minor modifications. First it could be restricted to in vivo situations, because the tissue inducing biomaterial cannot be carried out in vitro. So I think in vivo could appear in the term. And another minor modification is that eventually the tissue-induced biomaterials have also still involved but with no external living cells. So there are two modification. One is to restrict to in vivo, the other is "without addition of any external living cells."
Wei Sun	I always want to reduce the words. I think if we can get rid of "any" without addition of "living cells," then adding "and/or growth factor." But first of all, I support this. I think this represents

a new direction, new area of material. Get rid of, delete "any," and "and/or."

Nicholas Peppas	Dr. Sun, I don't understand why we have to remove the word "any." I do not think it has the meaning of "any possible living cell." I think it has the meaning of "whatever you present me, we'll work with it."
David Williams	Okay, thank you Nick.
Cato Laurencin	I think it's a great concept. It is a next generation concept, and I think that Professor Zhang's work in this has been really spectacular. Even in certain centers, the dogma is that you cannot regenerate without a morphogen, you cannot take stem cells and have regeneration occur without a morphogenetic protein to make the difference. And Professor Zhang was the first to counter that dogma, and say, No, you do not need a morphogen. The material itself, in the proper environment, can cause regeneration. And that change in dogma allows one to think in a revolutionary way, about how one can regenerate complex tissues. So absolutely I think it's an important term.
Carl Simon	Does it exclude drugs? Because it says living cells and growth factors, but what about drugs? Would it exclude drugs?
Kai Zhang	Yes I think so. No drugs.
Carl Simon	So should we mention drugs in that list?
Xingdong Zhang	No drugs. These materials can collect endogenous cell and endogenic growth factors.
Carl Simon	So another option, instead of listing everything that it does not include, just to be saying something like "only biomaterial properties" or something like that. Then somebody will say, "Well, what about a peptide," or, I do not know, somebody comes up something else. No genes, or something, I don't know, I am just trying to make the definition work. I know you wanted to focus on the materials, so maybe could change it to say "only the material properties required."
David Williams	I understand that, Carl. I think the definition is not too long to accommodate those. I think with this new concept the importance is to make it clear that you do not need those. But I do not think we have to be totally exhaustive on that one.
Kam Leong	I suggest replacing the first three words with just "biomaterials."
David Williams	Professor Zhang, any comments to remove the first two words? "Appropriately designed to start up with materials."
Kai Zhang	Okay.
David Williams	Kam, you okay with that?
Kam Leong	Well I don't really … Design is difficult. I just thought it would be cleaner, just use the word "biomaterials."

David Williams	I think the word "biomaterials" should be there, rather than material. I think the word "design" is there to try to convey the point that this is being specifically designed for that purpose, not just accidentally happens.
Kam Leong	That I could accept and now agree, but the first word should be "biomaterial."
David Williams:	Okay.
David Williams	Rena.
Rena Bizios	What is Kam asking? To substitute the word "appropriately" with something else? Or remove it completely?
Kam Leong	With the first three words, David said, keep the "design" in this one, and change the second word to "biomaterials."
Kai Zhang	Biomaterial.
Kam Leong	But anything specific-
David Williams	Yes you can. And when I made that point early yesterday morning, I said there are exceptions. And those exceptions are where you have more than one word in the title, and you simply can't avoid it.
Rena Bizios	I like your explanation, David, that this . . . There needs some word there about the design because it has to contrast the fact that we do not have anything else there. And it is a very specific plan and execution of a particular plan. So I thought that perhaps we should try to find a different word than "appropriately" that is not the right word. But I do not have a suggestion along those lines.
James Anderson	I have two comments. One is I think you should replace "could" by "can."
David Williams	Agreed from the English point of view.
James Anderson	Secondly, if you're going to include drugs, then you should include cytokines, and I could give you a list of other things that should be included. Drugs are not necessarily exclusive. I think that if you want to put in something additionally here, you might want to put in growth factors and other proliferative agents.
David Williams	Maybe, but I think that's getting a little bit too specific.
James Anderson	Well I think including drugs is exclusive.
Laura Poole-Warren	I think you could potentially have "without external addition of living cells and bioactive factors," which might cover all evils. And rather than "designed biomaterials" because I do not like the use of "design" as an adjective; it is a bit weird. "Biomaterials designed to regenerate damaged tissues and organs without external. . ."
David Williams	I like both of those, Laura. Wait a moment, let us get those down first.
Laura Poole-Warren	The first comment was to switch around, instead of having "designed biomaterials," "biomaterials designed to." "Designed to induce regeneration of damaged tissue."

Rui Reis	I consider the "damaged tissues or organs" part. I would take "organs" out, because I do not see an example of a biomaterial that is able to regenerate organs.
Laura Poole-Warren	Skin is an organ.
Cato Laurencin	Bone is an organ.
David Williams	I think you need "and/or" there. Yes. Rui, you heard what Cato said? That bone is an organ.
Rui Reis	Bone, okay. But does everybody consider bone as an organ here?
Laura Poole-Warren	And skin is an organ.
Rui Reis	Skin is an organ, but there is no biomaterial that regenerates skin.
Kam Leong	But the definition is tissue-inducing biomaterials, maybe it could be replaced to "tissue and organ induce."
David Williams	For a new concept, let us leave tissues and organs in. We can perhaps come back on another occasion, but leave them in for completeness.
Hua Ai	So besides damaged tissues or organs, I do not know if missing tissues, organs should be included or not?
David Williams	Hua's saying include "missing" as well as "damaged."
Wei Sun	I think damaged is easy enough, because damaged include trauma, injury and disease-caused injury, so it's enough. Damaged is okay.
Wei Sun	Also, may I suggest in biomaterial, the decision to induce regeneration of damaged tissue, that would be better.
Brendan Harley	One other maybe small wordsmithing thing, the "without external addition of living cells," one question is does that mean dead cells are okay? My suggestion might be "without addition of exogenous cells or bioactive factors" because the point is that external could be unclear as to what we mean.
David Williams	All agree on "exogenous" in there?
David Williams	That is good. "Exogenous" rather than "living." Kai, you okay with that?
Gouping Chen	I still think materials "bioactive" is difficult. So how about remove the "bioactive"? Because the material is bioactive. So it is better to change the bioactive word for other word.
David Williams	But I think the idea is this is the addition of, not the intrinsic characteristics. I think so. Okay. Yes?
Arthur Coury	For elegance, decide on your singular or plural.
David Williams	I think plural.
Arthur Coury	Then you should make it plural in the text.
David Williams	Sorry, what were you saying, Art?
Arthur Coury	Biomaterials.

David Williams	Oh, I see. But the phrase we are defining is "biomaterial," and I think normally we keep it as singular in the term.
Arthur Coury	I understand, but the title and the text were different.
David Williams	Okay, I understand.
William Wagner	I am not so clear on exogenous if your definition of the biomaterial incorporates encapsulated growth factors. I assume that is part of your biomaterial, but is that exogenous? Or if you have decellularized tissue and it has residual bioactive factors, that is intrinsic to that scaffold, so that is okay? I am just not clear on what is being added where and when and, what qualifies and what doesn't. I think it is a very important distinction.
David Williams	And so your specific question is? Remove exogenous?
William Wagner	No I think just cells.
David William	Without addition of cells and/or bioactive factors. All okay with that?
John Brash	To note that you have all three words there in the title are also in the definition; is that a concern.
David Williams	No, as I said before, I think if you've got a phrase which is more than one word, it's inevitable you're going to include one or more of those in the definition. One or more, I said. It is unusual to have all, I agree, but I do not know a way around that in this case.
Rena Bizios	I think we need to bring in the word "in vivo" and because this is only going to be achievable in vivo. So perhaps "biomaterials designed to induce in vivo the regeneration of damaged tissues."
David Williams	Kai, is that the concept, it has to be in vivo?
James Anderson	I have never heard of in vitro damaged tissues.
David Williams	No, but I think the question was, is there any parts of process which is in vitro? Like in a bioreactor.
Kai Zhang	I think this regeneration is quite clear. That probably indicates it is in vivo.
David Williams	It is clear, implied, so we do not need to include in the definition.
Kai Zhang	Yes, you do not need it.
David Williams	I am agreeing with that. So, for the moment, let us assume it is implied. Bill, you wanted to come back on that?
William Wagner	To clarify again, the best example of a tissue-induced biomaterial to my mind is decellularized tissue, which is bioactive, or functional, because it incorporates intrinsic bioactive factors. So when you look at that definition for decellularized matrices, it is a bit awkward. But it is a tissue-inducing biomaterial, right?
David Williams	Yes.
William Wagner	I think it is arguably one of the best tissue-inducing biomaterials. You are not adding anything, but it says "without" … Is it "designed"? So are these only synthetic materials, or are these

	natural materials? And if they are natural materials, where do you draw the line between bioactive factors and intrinsic factors?
David Williams	I agree with everything you said there, Bill. I think what we have to do is to say, have we got a definition good enough to start the concept in the lexicon, and that is going to be refined with further examples. My feeling is that this definition now is probably good enough for us to consider. And the text will say this is the first time this term is being defined. We can come back.
William Wagner	One potential workaround is just "biomaterials that induce the regeneration" so we can get rid of the "designed" and then it could make it more amendable to the decellularized matrix, or matrices that someone designed, or somewhere half way in the middle.
David Williams	We put "designed" in to ensure we're not talking about accidental effects. Or which just happens. Sorry?
Cato Laurencin	I guess instead of "addition," can we just use terms that are true to Professor Zhang's vision on this "without containing cells and/or bioactive factors." And I make that differentiation because I do not think that taking an allograft would not be a tissue-induced biomaterial. Fresh frozen allograft is a tissue-inducing biomaterial. It's already got cells. It's got factors in it, and you can take that fresh frozen allograft and put in that area.
Cato Laurencin	But we're thinking about biomaterials that are designed that actually do not contain cells or bioactive factors, and so a fresh frozen allograft would not be in that group. So to say "without containing cells and/or biological factors." Again, a freeze-dried matrix that still has bioactive factors would not be a tissue-inducing biomaterial because it's designed to function.
David Williams	Bill, does that include decellularized then?
William Wagner	No, because it is a biomaterial that induces tissue, so you are excluding one of the best biomaterials that induces tissue in that definition.
William Wagner	I would make the argument just to take out the "addition" Why do we care that you cannot add cells and bioactive factors? A tissue-inducing biomaterial, with our definition of biomaterial, why are we worried about this. "Cells," I get, but why are we worried about adding factors, chemicals, molecules that help with the induction? That's part of a biomaterial.
David Williams	I hear the concept is essentially the biomaterial does it itself.
Cato Laurencin	Without any biological factors involved.
William Wagner	So then why aren't we saying "purely synthetic materials," and say "tissue-inducing synthetic biomaterials"? Because our definition of biomaterial includes decellularized matrices, which quite a bit of inherent bioactivity. As well as natural matrices.

David Williams	Sure, but that is still the biomaterial, which is bioactive, doing it itself. This is without any addition.
William Wagner	It is a tissue-inducing biomaterial.
Kai Zhang	David? So I think the term is "tissue-inducing biomaterial," so probably the idea is really purely on the synthetic biomaterial. So instead of saying "biomaterial designed," we can say "synthetic biomaterial design."
David Williams	I can see that is where you came from, but Bill has a very important point. Maybe the best tissue-inducing biomaterial is decellularized tissue, we cannot exclude that from this new area.
Brendan Harley	I think maybe this is as close as we can get, because there can be some arguments about what constitute an added bioactive factor. There could be innate, the collagen scaffolds used in skin regeneration have charged proteoglycans that are mixed in there, and they do tons in terms of growth factors. So I think we can just leave it like this and say it is the definition.
Joachim Kohn	I would like to endorse what you said. For me, to simple minded, the word "addition" means that I take the biomaterial and I add stuff into it that was not there before. But if I take extracellular matrix and it already has stuff in it, it's actually fine. So the point I want to make is, this definition I think is as good as it gets. And I feel that we should just support it.
David Williams	Fine, I am liking that.
Peter Ma	Yes, so I also agree. This is where we are. There could be other things there - even you think of tooth as a material, we did not add growth factors or anything, but there could be calcium. Those things actually act on osteoblasts and others. Not an additional biological factor, but the materials have certain properties that can trigger them. So I guess that is potentially open for some other biomaterials as well.
Mário Barbosa	Very quickly, my suggestion is to remove the word "damaged" because we are excluding missing tissues.
David Williams	Kai? How important is damaged to you rather than just tissues? It is a good point.
Kai Zhang	Well we hope to include "damaged." Damage includes many different conditions. It can be trauma or injury related.
David Williams	So you are saying damage is not necessary?
Kai Zhang	No.
David Williams	It is?
Kai Zhang	It is necessary.
David Williams	Fine I thought that, yes. Okay, I think we have had enough discussion, a very good discussion.
David Williams	I agree with that, I was probably going to do it editorially, but I agree. If you can hyphenate, issue dash inducing.

James Anderson	David, before you vote, let me make a comment about what our colleague made here, and let's not forget, congenital deformities, those are not damaged tissues, they are missing tissues. This is where tissue-inducing biomaterials I think would play a very significant role. And you should consider including damaged or missing tissues or organs.
David Williams	Okay, anybody disagree with adding missing? We've been around a few times.
Arthur Coury	I would have to say though that is generating, it is not regenerating, so you might have to put that in. Let us have good English.
David Williams	We have all had a mild problem with what regeneration means, with a yes there I think we're happy with that. I do not know if we want to get into the difference between generate and regenerate. Let us leave it like that. I am seeing or hearing, that we include "missing" as well as "damaged." I think I got to close discussion there.
David Williams:	Fine, all happy with that? Professor Zhang, your expression is now in our dictionary, and in the field. Congratulations. Can you read this for me?

(d) Final Definition and Voting for Tissue-Inducing Biomaterial

Tissue-Inducing Biomaterial

A biomaterial designed to induce the regeneration of damaged or missing tissues or organs without the addition of cells and/or bioactive factors

Voting Yes	41
Voting No	6
Abstain	0
Total Votes	47
Number voting Yes or No	47
Percentage Yes Votes	87.2%

The definition achieved Consensus, having more than 75% Yes votes, with absolute number greater than 30.

G Other Biomaterials Types: No Voting, With or Without Discussion

A small number of terms were scheduled for discussion and voting during Session I but time allowed for only limited discussion and no votes were taken. The terms were "biomimesis" and its synonym "biomimicry," together with the biomaterial type "bioinspired material." The delegates were also offered a suggested definition of "biocomposite," but there was no enthusiasm to do so.

(a) Possible Definitions of "Biomimesis" and "Bioinspired Material" Included in Final Program

Biomimesis (Synonymous with Biomimicry)
Utilization of knowledge of the formation, structure or function of biologically produced substances or of biological processes, for the purpose of designing similar substances or processes by artificial means
Bioinspired Material
Synthetic material whose structure, properties or function mimics those of natural materials or living matter

(b) David Williams; Perspectives on "Biomimesis" and "Bioinspired Material" and Suggested Definition

David Williams	Biomimesis is the "utilization of knowledge of the formation, structure or function of biologically produced substances for the purpose of designing similar substances or processes by artificial means." And I say this is synonymous with "biomimicry." And a "bio-inspired material," is "a synthetic material whose structured properties or function mimics those of natural materials or living matter."

(c) Edited Discussion of "Biomimesis and Bioinspired Material"

Helen Lu	I have a question about the bioinspired versus biomimetic systems, if we can go to that slide, I will give a comment on that. To me, these two definitions are about the same thing. I think Kam Leong and I tried to do this together when we were talking about "bioinspired" versus "biomimetic." I think, for me, sometimes "bioinspired" has a different meaning, but the way the definition is right now, I feel that they are about the same thing.
David Williams	Yes, I tend to agree. Here, I was looking at the usage of these terms in the literature, and you will see, in fact, that "biomimesis" refers to a phenomenon; a "bioinspired material" is a noun. There is a difference there; that is why it is in that form. So, "biomimesis" is a generic utilization of knowledge. A "bioinspired material" is what is the outcome. I have to say, I am not a great fan of either of these terms or their meaning, but they are widely used. That is why I think we have to define them. Do you have an alternative suggestion?
Helen Lu	I was thinking "biomimetic materials" versus "bioinspired" because bioinspired, in some ways, you think about something that is used in nature, but in the real world, or the human world, we use it for something else. So, is it sort of an out-of-the-box use of a biological phenomenon or functionality, and biomimetic you really, especially for tissue engineering, you are mimicking nature in a

	way. So, I would suggest to maybe modify the definition to maybe defining biomimetic materials versus biomimesis.

David Williams   If we have these both as nouns, are you saying there is, or is not, a difference between a biomimetic material and a bioinspired material?

Helen Lu   I think, in terms of general biomaterial category, I would say the biomimetic materials would be more relevant than defining the process of mimicking nature. I think with the bioinspired I would change it to biomimetic. That would be my suggestion.

There were no further contributions to this discussion and no vote was taken.

IV

Biocompatibility and immune responses to biomaterials

Discussed in Session II and Final General Session

Session II Plenary Presentation: *James Anderson*
Session II Moderato: *Andrés García*
Session II Reporter: *Serena Best*
Final Session Moderator: *David Williams*
Final Session Reporters: *Carl Simon, Helen Lu, Serena Best*

A Biocompatibility

(a) Possible Definitions of "Biocompatibility" Included in Final Program

The ability of a material to perform with an appropriate host response in a specific application

(b) James Anderson; Perspectives on "Biocompatibility" and Suggested Definition

James Anderson   Let us begin with the first definition, "biocompatibility," which is found on page 13 of your booklet. This definition has served us well since Chester. This definition is internationally used. It is used by regulatory agencies. It will continue to be used by regulatory agencies. It will be continued to be used by colleagues working in the field of biomaterials. And no suggestion of change is made.

(c) Edited Discussion of "Biocompatibility"

Andrés García   Any discussions? Okay, if not, we are going to take the first vote, are we ready?

Definitions of Biomaterials for the Twenty-First Century
DOI: https://doi.org/10.1016/B978-0-12-818291-8.00004-3

(d) Final Definition and Voting for "Biocompatibility"

Biocompatibility

The ability of a material to perform with an appropriate host response in a specific application

Voting Yes	46
Voting No	1
Abstain	0
Total Votes	47
Number voting Yes or No	47
Percentage Yes Votes	97.9%

The definition achieved Consensus, having more than 75% Yes votes, with absolute number greater than 30.

B Inflammation

Editor's Note: A wide-ranging discussion took place in Session II around the broad subject of inflammation, with many comments, not surprisingly, involving the mechanisms and phenomena of immunity, hypersensitivity, and fibrosis. The most relevant comments from contributors are included in those sections judged to be most appropriate. In Session II, the resulting vote was inconclusive; a further discussion took place during the Final General Summary Session, and a further vote was taken. These two discussions are included here in Part One and Part Two respectively.

(a) Possible Definitions of "Inflammation" Included in Final Program

1. The immediate response by blood cells to injury/implantation/injection; initially acute inflammation (polymorphonuclear leukocytes) followed by chronic inflammation (monocytes, lymphocytes) with early resolution leading to the formation of granulation tissue surrounding the implant with subsequent fibrous capsule (fibrosis) formation and the foreign body reaction at the biomaterial/tissue interface
2. A localized tissue reaction, involving both cellular and humoral components, in response to infection, irritation or injury

(b) James Anderson; Perspectives on "Inflammation" and Suggested Definition

James Anderson   So innate immunity is inflammation, and what is inflammation? Inflammation is this series of events as it applies to biomaterials. It starts with acute inflammation; the continuum moves into chronic inflammation and into the formation of granulation tissue surrounding the implant and then subsequent fibrous capsule formation. And the foreign body reaction, consisting of macrophages and foreign body giant cells is seen at the biomaterial/tissue interface. This is acute inflammation, which is generally accepted in the biomaterials community.

(c) Edited Discussion of "Inflammation"

PART ONE: Discussion in Session II

Rena Bizios	I love all these definitions and they are very thorough and very up to the point. We need one definition for immunomodulation, because it has become a buzzword and no one knows what it means, especially the students. Going back to your definition of inflammation, and since we are focusing it on materials, should we put the foreign body reaction first before the encapsulation? In terms of the sequence of events. You know better than that, but I always think that foreign body reaction proceeds, or should proceed. Correct me if I am wrong.
James Anderson	I do not understand what your issue is.
Rena Bizios	You have presented the order of events that take place. And first we have the neutrophils and monocytes, macrophages. Then the granulation tissue formation and then as far as materials, interaction with materials, do the foreign body reaction events that precede the fibrous encapsulation formation. Therefore the order of appearance should be the subsequent foreign body reaction then fibrous capsule formation.
James Anderson	As we know, but is not included in this meeting, there is the classic Vroman effect, which involves protein adsorption to surfaces. And it to this surface that monocytes then adhere.
Andrés García	Another question is whether you should reverse the order of fibrosis and foreign body reaction.
James Anderson	I have no problem with that.
Helen Lu	Jim, I have a question about macrophages. You know there is a lot of literature on this, and people are working on studies where you differentiate monocytes into M1 or M2 macrophages, so I was wondering where you think would be a good place to put macrophages. Is it in inflammation or should we mention that here, or you want to have a separate term.
James Anderson	Macrophages form in two different areas, when we are considering implants. The first area, which is not commonly considered, is the surgical incision site, which starts to heal. That from my view and experience, plays virtually no role in terms of what is happening at the interface with the biomaterial. That is where monocytes adhere and start their differentiation process into macrophages. I will also tell you, that in my experience, I have seen no evidence of human monocyte proliferation. But we know that it does occur in rodents. And is misinterpreted by people using rodents for their basic research study. I urge caution until we have further evidence, but I

	have not seen it. Although there are people who are pushing the proliferation of monocytes in rodent species. So one has to be careful with this type of approach.
James Anderson	So it is the adherent monocytes, which actually occur virtually at the same time, that the acute inflammation is resolving. And monocytes are much more long-lived than leukocytes. So leukocytes die off, and you are left with the monocyte on the surface which, depending on what the current characteristics of that surface are, start the differentiation process.
Helen Lu	I agree with that.
Andrés García	Jim has a section on macrophages that he is commenting on later.
Helen Lu	Okay, so that is going to be discussed. I was not sure if we should mention it here in the inflammation process.
Hua Ai	Jim, it is a good definition, I only have a small suggestion. You mentioned implant, and also the biomaterial tissue interface, and so in the first sentence, I think it is okay to be general. We have injury, implantation and injection, but for this biomaterials definition, I think maybe you just put "implantation/injection."
James Anderson	I should put "implantation"?
Hua Ai	Only "implantation and injection." Remove "injury."
James Anderson	I disagree. The extent and degree of injury determines the extent and degree of inflammation. And it is good to remind the user of this definition that there are different types of injury.
Mário Barbosa	Jim, the formation of a fibrous capsule is not common to every implantable material. If you are using a material that degrades, you don't have the formation of a fibrous capsule. I wonder whether a reference to foreign body reaction, without mentioning fibrous capsule or fibrous capsule formation, in all cases, will be more correct.
Mário Barbosa	Formation. Because if the material degrades you do not have the formation of fibrous capsule.
James Anderson	If the material is not there?
Mário Barbosa	If the material is not there. Because it has degraded, you do not have the formation of a fibrous capsule.
James Anderson	With a degradable polymer?
Mário Barbosa	Yes.
James Anderson	Not necessarily true. Yes, you agree.
Mário Barbosa	But your definition is general in the sense you admit there is always fibrous capsule formation, which is not naturally true.
James Anderson	I have a definition for fibrous capsule formation, which will be forthcoming. But once you form the fibrous capsule, the fibrous capsule will undergo the process of remodeling. And the fibrous capsule thickness is dependent upon the chemical characteristics of

the material. Hydrophilic materials have a thinner fibrous capsule than hydrophobic materials. We do not understand why, but that is the data.

James Anderson	The process of remodeling does several things, and we have several definitions that we can get to later. But it condenses the collagen in the fibrous capsule and in that process, which you see is a thinner but denser fibrous capsule, that collagen degradation enzymes come into play and also reduce the fibrous capsule surrounding the material.
Andrés García	Mario, are you proposing an amendment to this definition?
James Anderson	It is important to look at this in the context of your specific system and make a determination as to what components have an interplay in your specific material or medical device.
Arthur Coury	I would make two comments. With our biodegradable hydrogels, we would form a fibrous capsule and have apple jelly underneath until it went away. And you would have some sort of a scar at the end of it. But the other thing, Jim, having to do with timing and again, it is experience but not expertise here. My understanding was the first thing to really deposit on an implant was a monocyte, and it would attract the PMNs. So in terms of timing, I wonder if it is better to use the word "dominant" rather imply the very first thing are PMNs.
James Anderson	We have done studies in the cage implant system and this is ultimately what we see. After the first week, because the polymorphonuclear leukocytes have a finite lifetime, in fact, they're probably dead and the debris is undergoing phagocytosis within the first couple of days. Monocytes being more long-lived, then become the predominant cell type at the surface.
James Anderson	We do not make a distinction there. I did not want to make a distinction.
Arthur Coury	The term "initially," that is what I was addressing.
Maria J. Vicent	I like the terms in general, but for this one, "inflammation," it is difficult. Not all biomaterials are considered implants, so for those that are not implants, this definition may be restricting. Maybe we can make it broader, and the part of the formation of granulation tissues around the implant could be amplified for, just in the case that it is an implant, this is happening. Magnesium, for example, a biomaterial used in the blood circulation, and it is acting there, but is not generating a fibrosis capsule. We should considering making a definition broader for those biomaterials not used as implants.
James Anderson	In my experience, natural materials are not implanted. I say that because chitosan type materials, collagen type materials, and other materials prepared from natural polymers have all undergone a modification procedure. They have all undergone a fabrication

	procedure. They have a different level of organization. So to use the term natural, is not correct.
Andrés García	Were you referring to materials that go in the bloodstream?
Maria J. Vicent	Exactly, I am working with polypeptides. Polypeptides are administered in the blood and they can act at the blood level. They do not form a capsule even if they are involved in an inflammation reaction. As these types of biomaterial are not implants, so I was just suggesting to maybe make the definition a bit broader. To consider also those types of situations, where we do not have implants and therefore we do not have a capsule formation. We are working with biomaterials, but not as implants.
James Anderson	A biomaterial that is not an implant? Then it is not a biomaterial, is it? Like what, a stent?
Maria J. Vicent	No, no, like a nanoparticle or nanogel, that goes in the blood circulation.
James Anderson	Injection. How do you introduce a nanoparticle?
Maria J. Vicent	With an injection, then you do not have a capsule, for example.
David Williams	Jim, not surprising I do have a few problems here. One relates to what Maria was trying to mention. You do refer to implant, and when looking at biomaterials, there are many applications of biomaterials other than implants. I am thinking of a tissue engineering scaffold, for example, where inflammation becomes a major issue; it is not implanted and there's no fibrous capsule.
David Williams	Secondly, I have some problem with the time sequence, the temporal issues here. You well know, Jim, when you have biodegradable polymers, you do have initial acute inflammation, you have chronic inflammation, which resolves or subsides, and at a later stage, which can be a few years later, then re-stimulates inflammation. It is not, in my opinion, a simple transition from acute to chronic inflammation and resolution. I think we have to encompass that temporal sequence.
James Anderson	Yes, but what you have described is a specific example dealing with a specific type of polymer with specific characteristics. This definition may change with that. This is the simplest definition that we have for the implantation of a device.
Rena Bizios	I would like to propose a friendly amendment. "Blood cells to tissue injury" take that "slash" out and "biomaterial implantation/injection or implantation/injection of biomaterials." Because we separate the two and perhaps things will fall into place a little bit better.
James Anderson	You're suggesting putting tissue engineering in?
Rena Bizios	No, I said tissue injury, not engineering. Tissue injury and then the implantation/injection is associated with the materials of the implant device, something along the lines.

James Anderson	Yes, but then that also comes back to the previous comment, where blood is considered a tissue.
Rena Bizios	It was prompted by that comment, in terms of perhaps making it something that will cover that particular comment as well.
James Anderson	I do not have a problem putting that in as an insert. If it is the group's desire.
Andrés García	So if I can circle back, what I have heard, the discussion centers around whether we have this persistent fibrous encapsulation of whether the material is implanted or whether the material goes into the bloodstream for example. Or as David alluded to, would be degraded and replaced by tissue. I think that is where the crux of the discussion is. Right, David?
Laura Poole-Warren	Just looking at some of these definitions, they are very much out there in other fields and often driven by other fields and perhaps we need to nuance them for biomaterials. However, "inflammation" is one that seems to me, is one that we perhaps do not need to play with too much, because I think it has been around for a long time and I think it still covers the fact that a foreign body is introduced and the foreign body could be a biomaterial. I think we are trying to reinvent a wheel that we perhaps do not need to reinvent. I would like to pick up on Maria's comment on contact and I think if we look at the FDA definitions of the nature of contact, they are very definitely indirect and direct contacts that are not necessarily implantable.
Laura Poole-Warren	For example, contact lenses. They are not an implant as such, they're actually on the surface. There are many devices that are actually on the surface of the skin and are not classically considered implants.
James Anderson	I would take argument with that point. I have seen foreign body giant cells overgrowing contact lenses.
Laura Poole-Warren	There can be inflammation, absolutely. But the device is not an implant.
William Wagner	I will jump on the train here and say extracorporeal devices, oxygenators, et cetera, where you have activation of immune cells in an inflammatory response that shows up in other tissues, but don't ultimately get encapsulated. And then the other question is, is complement activation part of the inflammatory response, I would argue it is, but this says, "immediate response by blood cells." And I would say, in some cases, there is humoral activation that triggers it.
Xingdong Zhang	I agree with the content but this definition is too long. We can leave only the important parts.
David Williams	I agree with that. I think it does look long. I do not know, bearing in mind my comment, that we should not get into discussions of mechanisms. I am not sure we need to mention cell types in this.

As I mentioned, I think we have to be a little careful about the temporal sequence, the timing. My suggestion would be, for example, take out "immediate." The response by blood cells, and as Bill said, maybe humoral systems. I think you should say through injury, however caused. And then take out the reference to blood cells and then take out the reference to surrounding implant. As Laura said, there are circuits which trigger inflammation and there's no fibrous capsule.

David Williams   My suggestion is, this is a good basis for a definition. Perhaps we need to discuss this a bit offline and come back tomorrow afternoon with a slightly refined and shortened version of this, which encompasses the point you are trying to make, Jim, but is a bit less unwieldy.

Maria J. Vicent   I would suggest, just to delete the sentence, "the formation of granulation tissues surround the implant with subsequent fibrous capsule formation" and... I would delete that sentence. And then I would leave the rest, it might make sense.

James Anderson   We can follow David's suggestion. Well Rena had a comment.

Rena Bizios   I have to ask all of you to keep in mind who the audience of these definitions is going to be. I am an educator and I teach biomaterials every semester. Therefore, when I give this to the students, I bring to them two things. First of all, that we have to distinguish between what happens in nature or in physiology, what blood cells do to tissue injury. And then what has happened around the implant. And I like them to have from the very beginning, in their minds, that there is a sequence of events and they should be prepared to see what these events are and how to describe these events and what happens. So from my perspective, I like this longer definition.

James Anderson   At this point, what we would like to do is to vote this definition. To see where we are. And then we will have a second vote. But let us vote this first.

Andrés García   Okay, we're going to take a vote on what is on the screen now.

Andrés García   Okay, I think we have most of the votes, and it is clear that it is not approved. So we will revise the definition.

James Anderson   Yes. Now discussion is done. David has made an amendment, which I do not completely understand but would you communicate with our reporter as to what you think this should be changed to? And let's understand that what we are talking about are general definitions. They can be applied to specific examples, where processes like these, in a continuum... And that's the important thing to remember. That this is a continuum, change. We may have no fibrous capsule at the end, depending on what the surface of the material is. Actually, what the surface of the device is. There may be changes in the different cellular compositions.

(d) Final Definition and Voting for "Inflammation"

Inflammation

The immediate response by blood cells to injury/implantation/injection; initially acute inflammation (polymorphonuclear leukocytes) followed by chronic inflammation (monocytes, lymphocytes) with early resolution leading to the formation of granulation tissue surrounding the implant with subsequent fibrous capsule (fibrosis) formation and the foreign body reaction at the biomaterial/tissue interface

Voting Yes	18
Voting No	27
Abstain	2
Total Votes	47
Number voting Yes or No	45
Percentage Yes Votes	40%

The definition achieved neither consensus nor provisional consensus.

PART TWO: Discussion in Final Session

Editor's Note: Following the discussions in Session II, several delegates tried to come up with a modified definition that could be discussed again. The following is the preferred option that arose.

Inflammation/Innate Immunity
The immune response to injury and the implantation or injection of a biomaterial. This cascade comprises contact activation with blood cells and humoral factors, acute inflammation, and chronic inflammation, with resolution either leading to fibrous capsule (fibrosis) formation at the biomaterial/tissue interface or tissue remodeling

Andrés García	Again, Jim yesterday indicated that innate immunity, we are going to treat equivalently to inflammation, and that is the proposed definition. "The immune response to injury, and the implantation or injection of a biomaterial," and then discussing a general sequence of events, we are at the humoral factors I think Bill brought up, then we had a long discussion as to whether you had the end result as fibrosis. I think that the wording at the end is from Mario that the resolution is either this fibrosis, or tissue remodeling in the event at the implant is fully degraded.
James Anderson	There were two changes that we made earlier today. I think you said we were going to include "innate" in front of "immune." Then, one other change is fibrous capsule formation and at the biomaterial tissue interface ... and tissue remodeling. It's not an "or," it's "and tissue remodeling." You have to have tissue there before you can remodel it. Right at the bottom.

Andrés García	I thought, Jim, that we were keeping fibrous capsule with the understanding that fibrosis involves tissue remodeling. The second part is to address when the implant is no longer persisting, and the capsule ends up getting remodeled.
David Williams	I think that's very helpful. I have one comment, Jim. There are some situations where there is no resolution, where in fact you end up with chronic tissue damage, as in the metal on metal hips.
James Anderson	Then that is an inadequate and inappropriate device or material. Period.
David Williams	It is still inflammation, isn't it?
James Anderson	No, it's … no, no, in fact with this specific example you're using, is a … type four hypersensitivity reaction.
David Williams	I understand that, but what about the biodegradable, PLLA materials, which had late stage degradation, which involved very significant inflammation, three or four years later, and serious chronic tissue damage.
James Anderson	No, no, there's not chronic damage. When you inject those materials, they form a fibrous capsule where the foreign body reaction around the material, which ultimately degrades the material, leading to fibrosis, which undergoes remodeling.
David Williams	I wasn't referring to injecting, I was referring to maxillofacial fracture plates, which are implanted, and three or four years later, it was serious chronic inflammation, and tissue damage, and they had to be removed.
Cato Laurencin	I would argue that that was an additional insult that prompts a new series of acute to chronic inflammation. Either the introduction of wear particles is a new insult and injury that starts inflammation over, or the degradation products then start a new injury and insult that starts acute and chronic inflammation. It is not that the original inflammation cascade did not happen, it is this is a new injury.
David Williams	I agree with that. That is what we're here for. At the end of that day, even it is a new one, that is still inflammation, isn't it?
Cato Laurencin	Yes, but it is a new event - it doesn't circumvent, it doesn't say this did not happen, it is just saying that is starts over.
David Williams	I agree, but my comment was meant to say, as well as having acute inflammation, and chronic inflammation with resolution, either leading to fibrous capsule formation at the bone interface, and tissue remodeling, I am saying there can be chronic tissue damage.
James Anderson	I am fine with that.
Laura Poole-Warren	I find the first part of this a bit repetitive. It is just saying what the actual term is. Innate immunity, it's the innate immune response, I would possibly suggest that we be a bit more specific, and say that it's a local, physiological response to tissue damage, and implantation or injection of a biomaterial. In essence, the second

	part is really nice because it does go through what happens with biomaterials. It would be nice to include, somehow, the fact that this is part of the normal physiological healing response. Now, of course, with biomaterials, it can go wrong. I am not quite sure how to include that, but I think it would be nice to actually have a nod to the fact that inflammation is actually a normal physiological response, and part of the healing response.
Arthur Coury	Can we leave out topical application here because you could have irritation right away, even if it is not a response of the innate immune system.
David Williams	Sorry, what are you suggesting to leave out?
Arthur Coury	I would not leave out topical application. It could even be for days that you apply something topically.
David Williams	You are suggesting implantation, or injection, or topical application? Let's go to Jim. You okay with that?
Laura Poole-Warren	You could actually just be very broad and say, "Contact with biomaterial," rather than all of those things.
James Anderson	The inflammation is a pathological response, not necessarily a physiological response. You do not study inflammation when you study physiology.
Laura Poole-Warren	No, no, I wasn't talking about that point. I was actually talking about the point relating to contact, which is "implantation, injection, or topical application," I was just simply suggesting that what we can do is, we can actually say, "Contact with biomaterial," whether it's direct or indirect.
William Wagner	I like it much better than yesterday. The one concern I have is the oxygenator, dialysis, extracorporeal device, where we study inflammatory pathway activation, the implications are serious for the patients in terms of pulmonary edema. It is a systemic effect, there is no encapsulation, there is complement activation, there is leukocyte activation, there are inflammatory pathways, but it is not leading to this. This is for implanted biomaterials, but not necessarily extracorporeal biomaterial content. I endorse that one. I think the problem with the definition is the encapsulation because it really narrows the definition.
David Williams	I agree with Bill.
William Wagner	That part.
David Williams	What are you suggesting?
William Wagner	Deleting just how it happens, because this is only happening by implants.
Andrés García	Sorry, if I understand, two things, Bill. You will get rid of "local," right? Then, Maria's point is, and the example that Bill gave is really the first part of that cascade.

David Williams	You could say at the end, and "in the case of implanted biomaterials, leading to fibrous..."
Andrés García	That is one way, what I was thinking is, could we say, "This cascade may comprise the three things," or no?
William Wagner	You get the contact activation, the blood cells, humoral factors, acute inflammation, all that's going on. The difference is that it is on a large scale, and it has systemic effects in other organ systems.
Andrés García	What you are saying, after factors, say in the case of an implant, or injection of material, you have this other one?
William Wagner	Yes, in the case of the implant, then I think this is all an important part of that completion of the inflammatory processes, fibrous encapsulation, remodeling, that is all very relevant for talking about inflammation in implants. In this other world of acute contact, usually acute, large surface area of contact, the implications are systemic.
Andrés García	I understand, but how do we construct that on the sentence? We break the sentence up into two or ... then we have a paragraph definition.
James Anderson	Well, it is important to note that the examples that Bill uses are downstream examples. They are not necessarily occurring at the point where these mechanisms are turned on. Whether it be dialyzer, an oxygenator, et cetera. Previously, we had a local response, and if that gets inserted back, then we are talking about implants, and what is happening right at the device.
David Williams	The implant.
James Anderson	Complement is activated on a dialysis membrane. It does not have its effect there. The effect is downstream.
David Williams	The point it, it is inflammation. It is biomaterial centered inflammation. The biomaterial has caused inflammation, and it is having an effect on the patient. If we define inflammation in the context of biomaterials, I think we need to address that aspect of it.
James Anderson	I do not believe we have to stress it, I think we could mention it. I appreciate where you come from, but I come from a different world.
David Williams	We are both in the biomaterials world.
Andrés García	David, do you have a recommendation on how to capture that?
David Williams	I knew it would come to this, Andrés. I thought of this all night. I understand exactly where Jim is, but we are talking here is about how inflammation is associated with an implanted device, which is primarily, not necessarily totally, but primarily local. Bill is absolutely right, there is another situation where we have primarily extracorporeal circulation, where the inflammatory effect is systemic. The question is, can we put both of those into the same definition, or do we have to separate these into two terms.

David Williams	I don't know exactly how to do that because unless we say, implant associated inflammation, and extracorporeal circulation associated inflammation. Does that make any sense?
William Wagner	If you let of the, "With resolution." I think it weakens it, but it makes it more generally applicable. The implant, you definitely have that, but that, I would argue, is more part of the foreign body response, and would be covered more in the definition of the foreign body response. Then, just leave it like that because, acute inflammation, if you're talking to a cardiac surgeon, they are going to worry about that after bypass grafting.
Andrés García	Bill, if we end the sentence after "chronic inflammation," and then say in the case of implantable ... whatever, materials ... something ... chronic inflammation may resolve ... resolving to fibrous capsule formation.
James Anderson	There may be a better way to say that. What Bill is talking about is ex vivo devices. Perhaps a sentence at the end, where we specify ex vivo devices ... may lead to ... downstream inflammatory effects.
Elizabeth Cosgriff-H	It could also be circulating, as well. It could also be circulating particles. If they circulate long enough, you could get systemic effects.
James Anderson	Well, yes, we understand that, but the examples that are being used are all ex vivo.
Elizabeth Cosgriff-H	Yes, but they don't have to be ex vivo, they could be circulating, and have the same effect.
James Anderson	No, they don't. They don't have to be.
David Williams	Can we just use systemic rather than downstream?
James Anderson	I am fine with that.
David Williams	We have the second part, after you have said "in the case of," we could have, "in the case of ex vivo devices ..."
James Anderson	"May lead to systemic inflammatory effects."
David Williams	I am not sure you're done, you have taken note in the case of implantable devices?
Andrés García	You want that?
David Williams	Can you go back? After chronic inflammation there, yes.
Andrés García	Sorry.
David Williams	"In the case of implantable devices"
Andrés García	That's not quite right.
David Williams	This may lead to ... yes, fine. "Lead to resolution," et cetera. Fine, and in the last one, "in the case of ex vivo devices, this may lead to systemic inflammatory effects." Andrés?
Andrés García	I am happy with that. Jim?
James Anderson	That's fine.

David Williams	Does that mean Jim, Andrés, and myself agree? Looks like.
David Williams	Any comments on that, then? Are we ready to try to vote on that?
Ruggero Bettini	Second sentence, start with this cascade, but the word cascade along the first line. Maybe we can say, "This response." Second sentence. Replace it with "response."
David Williams	Okay. Laura, you don't like that?
Laura Poole-Warren	No, it wasn't that. I am wondering with "implantation, injection, or topical application," does that cover ex vivo?
David Williams	No.
Laura Poole-Warren	You could just say, more broadly, "and contact with biomaterials." Is that too broad?
James Anderson	I am fine with that.
David Williams	I am fine with that, too.
Laura Poole-Warren	"Physiological response to injury and contact with biomaterial."
James Anderson	That first sentence doesn't make sense. It needs a verb.
Andrés García	Why don't we, can we get rid of this response, and just say, "this response . . . that comprises."
James Anderson	I think we are pretty close, David.
David Williams	Anybody want to comment on that? I think we should move on that.
David Williams	Should we just say, "A physiological response to injury . . . and contact with the biomaterial, the comprised activation," rather than including all the content there?
Andrés Garcia	I think that's fine. Just have activation. Okay.
David Williams	In the case of implant devices . . .. What's the suggestion?
David Williams	Yes. In the third line, this may lead to the formation, yes. It takes that resolution, though. Where do we lead, this may lead to resolution.
James Anderson	Resolves, it goes away.
Serena Best:	. . .in the formation, and resulting in. . .
Andrés García	We can say this process leads to either . . . No?
William Wagner	Why don't we just say, "This may lead to the formation of a fibrous capsule or chronic . . .." Yes, right.
Hua Ai	Yes, I think, "contact with" is a good word. It is broad. But compared to the original "implantation/injection," maybe it is kind of too mild in some cases. So, is that contact between the biomaterial and the tissue organ every case to generate this information, so.
David Williams	I think "contact" is okay. It is not ideal, but it avoids us having to put "inflammation" and an "ex vivo circuit" in the same phrase. Okay, I am inclined to leave it there. Okay last word Rena.
Rena Bizios	I think it requires a comma after "devices."

Andrés García   David, I assume that you will do some grammar checking of all the things. So I propose we vote on this. The commas can be added later.

(e) Final Definition and Voting for "Inflammation/Innate Immunity"

Editor's Note: As the above discussion shows, there was much comment on the final wording and syntax, such that the editor was asked to carry out some grammatical adjustments. The following definition arises from this:

Inflammation/Innate Immunity

The response to injury or contact with biomaterials, involving a cascade of events including activation with blood cells and humoral factors, and both acute and chronic inflammation. In the case of implanted devices this may lead to resolution with fibrous capsule formation and remodeling; with ex vivo devices, this may lead to systemic effects

Voting Yes	33
Voting No	13
Abstain	0
Total Votes	46
Number voting Yes or No	46
Percentage Yes Votes	71.7%

The definition achieved provisional consensus with over 50% Yes votes.

C Adaptive Acquired Immune System

(a) Possible Definitions of "Adaptive Acquired Immune System" Included in Final Program

Adaptive Immunity (synonymous with Acquired Immunity)
An immunological subsystem, characterized by memory, that provides protection from a pathogen or toxin, being mediated by B and T cells and highly specific to a given antigen

(b) James Anderson; Perspectives on "Adaptive Acquired Immune System" and Suggested Definition

James Anderson   The next topic that we will have is this issue of adaptive or the acquired immune system, and under this, we have hypersensitivity. And hypersensitivity is the classic definition, which is one, an abnormal sensitivity to an allergen, drug or other agent associated with an exaggerated immune response. From the biomaterials perspective, latex gloves are probably the best example and for the most part are no longer utilized clinically. The suggested definition is as follows:

Adaptive Acquired Immune System

The adaptive immune system consists of lymphocytes and their products, including antibodies. Humeral immunity is mediated by B (Bone marrow-derived) lymphocytes and their secreted products, antibodies (Immunoglobulins). Cellular immunity is mediated by T (Thymus-derived) lymphocytes and includes helper, cytotoxic and regulatory lymphocytes and natural killer cells

(c) Edited Discussion of "Adaptive Acquired Immune System"

There was no discussion of the adaptive acquired immune system apart from situations where this topic was included in dialogue concerning hypersensitivity.

(d) Final Definition and Voting for "Adaptive Acquired Immune System"

Adaptive Acquired Immune System

The adaptive immune system consists of lymphocytes and their products, including antibodies. Humeral immunity is mediated by B (Bone marrow-derived) lymphocytes and their secreted products, antibodies (Immunoglobulins). Cellular immunity is mediated by T (Thymus-derived) lymphocytes and includes helper, cytotoxic and regulatory lymphocytes and natural killer cells

Voting Yes	35
Voting No	7
Abstain	5
Total Votes	47
Number voting Yes or No	42
Percentage Yes Votes	83.3%

The definition achieved Consensus, having more than 75% Yes votes, with absolute number greater than 30.

(e) Further Commentary on the Definition of "Adaptive Acquired Immune System"

In the context that David Williams was given the authority to make minor grammatical alterations, a slightly better wording is as follows, avoiding repetition of the term within the definition and avoiding unnecessary explanations in the definition. It is this which is confirmed to have consensus:

Adaptive Acquired Immune System

A system consisting of lymphocytes and their products, including antibodies; humeral immunity is mediated by B lymphocytes and their secreted immunoglobulins and cellular immunity is mediated by T lymphocytes including helper, cytotoxic and regulatory lymphocytes and natural killer cells

D Hypersensitivity

(a) Possible Definitions of "Hypersensitivity" Included in Final Program

An abnormal sensitivity to an allergen, drug or other agent, associated with an exaggerated immune response

(b) James Anderson; Perspectives on "Hypersensitivity" and Suggested Definition

1) An abnormal sensitivity to an allergen, drug or other agent, associated with an exaggerated immune response.
2) Tissue injury immune reactions produced by four mechanisms:
    Type I – Immediate production of IgE antibody;
    Type II – Antibody Mediated, production of IgG and/or IgM;
    Type III – Immune Complex Mediated, deposition of antigen-antibody complexes
        with complement activation;
    Type IV – Cell Mediated, activation of T lymphocytes.

(c) Edited Discussion of "Hypersensitivity"

Timmie Topoleski	Just a question, Jim, to help me out. For number two, all four of those are not necessary for hypersensitivity, right. Is it one of the four? So it should produce by one of these four mechanisms, right.
Andrés García	Tim is proposing to decide on one of four mechanisms.
James Anderson	Well I would alter your suggestion and say by any of four, that's for clarity.
Timmie Topoleski	Okay, thank you.
Elizabeth Cosgriff-H	For these to distinguish that we are talking about immune responses to materials, would it help to change these, instead of saying "inflammation," saying "inflammatory response" or "hypersensitivity reaction" or "acquired immune response"? To indicate that we are trying to differentiate between the immunity versus immune response to a material.
James Anderson	Well we commonly talk about hypersensitivity reactions to materials. And they are identified by these possible mechanisms. And that is information that comes out of our testing procedures.
Elizabeth Cosgriff-H	And so I think just adding reaction, hypersensitivity reaction, immune response or inflammatory response to each of these would help clarify that these are responses to the materials.
James Anderson	Oh, you're just saying add reactions to hypersensitivity? That's fine.
Elizabeth Cosgriff-H	I was just saying the inflammatory and immune response.
James Anderson	David?
David Williams	Just so I am clear, are we saying in definition two, that one, two and three are all hypersensitivity responses? As well as four?

James Anderson	That is the classic physiologic definition. Yes. And any of them can occur. But I must say that I have yet to see examples of two and three. Two, I am not quite sure about because it has to do with vaccination. Which is a positive application or identification, but as I said, this is device and biomaterials specific. You apply this to what you have.
Rena Bizios	I know where you are coming from in terms of allergens and drugs, but should we make it a little more specific, add biomaterials or implants? The other agents specified bring the materials or the implants into the picture.
James Anderson	You are talking about number two?
Rena Bizios	No, no, number one. The end of the first line — "or other agent." Make it a biomaterial, make it an implant so it will bring in the material aspect of hypersensitivity.
James Anderson	Well, I described that in terms of leachables, redundant catalysts, which have all been worked over, depending upon what the medical device is, for example, catalysis of the silicone rubber with a breast implants. Those types of issues.
Andrés García	Okay, I think we reached the convergence point, so we are going to vote with these two minor amendments that Tim and Elizabeth have made, right.
Kai Zhang	Andrés, are you going to modify any of this or are you going to vote and then modify later, I am a little bit confused here.
James Anderson	Yes, we are going to make the modification that Elizabeth selected, was hypersensitivity reactions. Is it possible for us to make that change now and then vote?
Laura Poole-Warren	Could I just make a comment here. With the hypersensitivity reactions, it is not clear in the definition that these are actually acquired immune responses. So the acquired aspect is missing from that definition. Is that an oversight that we want to correct?
James Anderson	We will go back and look at that definition and if it needs the hypersensitivity to be put in, we definitely will put it in.
Laura Poole-Warren	Thank you.
James Anderson	Now, I want to make clear, that I am not sure that I have seen all these. But my target is the future. And when we get into sophisticated systems like scaffolds, with stem cells, and as David said, no fibrous capsule, which is incorrect. We're going to see these types of responses. If we do not see these types of responses, we have to be open to identifying these types of responses, because they ultimately may lead to a failure of the device.

Peter Ma	Maybe we will just vote on item one of the two. Because based on the rules in the beginning, it is not good to have mechanisms in the definition, if we all agree on that.
James Anderson	We can vote in multiple definitions and we are suggesting both of these as being definitions for a hypersensitivity reaction.
Andrés García	I have made the amendment, let us vote on this definition. If it doesn't pass, we can do further revisions to the definition, but we have a lot of stuff to cover. And I think the discussion is getting redundant.
Andrés García	So please open it up. So please vote on what is on the screen.

(d) Final Definition and Voting for "Hypersensitivity Reaction"

Hypersensitivity Reaction

Tissue injury immune reaction produced by one of four mechanisms:
Type I – Immediate production of IgE antibody;
Type II – Antibody Mediated, production of IgG and/or IgM;
Type III – Immune Complex Mediated, deposition of antigen-antibody complexes
with complement activation;
Type IV – Cell Mediated, activation of T lymphocytes

Voting Yes	37
Voting No	8
Abstain	2
Total Votes	47
Number voting Yes or No	45
Percentage Yes Votes	82.2%

The definition achieved Consensus, having more than 75% Yes votes, with absolute number greater than 30.

(e) Further Commentary on the Definition of "Hypersensitivity Reaction"

In the context that David Williams was given the authority to make minor grammatical alterations, a slightly better wording is as follows; this amendment was made since the definition as it stands does not refer to "acquired" and could be construed to encompass primary irritation. It is this which is confirmed to have consensus:

Hypersensitivity Reaction

Tissue injury acquired immune reaction produced by one of four mechanisms:
Type I – Immediate production of IgE antibody;
Type II – Antibody Mediated, production of IgG and/or IgM;
Type III – Immune Complex Mediated, deposition of antigen-antibody complexes
with complement activation;
Type IV – Cell Mediated, activation of T lymphocytes

E Myofibroblast

(a) Possible Definitions of "Myofibroblast" Included in Final Program

None was included as the term was not on the original list of terms to be discussed.

(b) James Anderson; Perspectives on "Myofibroblast" and Suggested Definition

James Anderson	Let us move to the next one then. Myofibroblasts. From my perspective, and in particular, my clinical perspective, myofibroblasts would appear to be playing a more important role when we consider scaffold-type materials. This is a cell type in the final healing phase, which has not generally been considered as a significant cell type. But there is evidence in the literature that myofibroblasts produce more collagen than fibroblasts.
James Anderson	Importantly, they contain alpha smooth muscle cell actin and are responsible for the contractility of scar tissue or, if you will, the fibrous capsule. More importantly, they have been identified in the liver and in the lung and in the kidney as being the primary cell type for fibrotic disease. Not the fibroblasts but the myofibroblasts.
James Anderson	And I would suspect that in the future, we are going to see and hear more about the myofibroblasts. In particular, the last sentence there, where it identifies myofibroblasts as "sensing and modulating extracellular matrix stiffness through focal adhesions."
James Anderson	There is one point I have not put in here. And that is the epithelial to mesenchymal cell transition. This is now well identified in the biological and clinical literature. And macrophages, and I do not like this word, but I will use it, macrophages in a sense de-differentiate and can come back as another cell type. This epithelial to mesenchymal cell translation, I think is going to be very important in the future.[1]
James Anderson	Now this may be an incomplete definition. But at least it provides a definition, which in the future, will probably be modified, depending upon information that is forthcoming. This at least identifies it within the book that will be produced as a cell type for consideration by investigators.

Suggested definition:

Myofibroblasts

Primary extracellular matrix (ECM) - secreting cells containing alpha-smooth muscle actin during wound healing and fibrosis and are responsible for the contractility of scar

---

[1] Williams DF, Biocompatibility pathways: Biomaterials-induced sterile inflammation, mechanotransduction, and principles of biocompatibility control, *ACS Biomaterials Sci Eng*, 2017, 3(1), 2–35.

tissue. Myofibroblast progenitors include resident fibroblasts, fibrocytes, pericytes and may also result from epithelial/endothelial to mesenchymal transition. Myofibroblasts sense and modulate ECM stiffness through focal adhesions via integrin binding

(c) Edited Discussion of "Myofibroblast"

Rena Bizios	The first sentence, the first phrase needs a verb to have parallel structure for the rest of the other two sentences. Primary extracellular matrix I would say "extracellular matrix - secreting cells" which are responsible for the contractility. Some little modification there.
Jiandong Ding	James, would you like to modify the presentation to make it like a definition instead of just some descriptions?
James Anderson	Is there a difference between description and definition? We are talking about a cell type, which has already been identified in the tissue response.
Jiandong Ding	So it is better to first give a very clear definition of what a myofibroblast is and then give some description of its function.
James Anderson	Well that's what the first sentence says is they secrete ECM containing smooth muscle actin. Do you have a recommendation? Specifically says what the cell type is and where it's found.
Jiandong Ding	Yes but in case it looks like a definition about ECM.
James Anderson	No I don't, the English says cells, secreting cells.
Arthur Coury	This is from Bill Wagner's work where I've heard people fighting and arguing as to whether the cells that he generates at the heart from a biomaterial after an infarction, smooth muscle cells or are they myofibroblasts. I am just wondering, does this description distinguish between the two types of cells. Smooth muscle cells versus myofibroblast. It is hard to see them microscopically as being different.
James Anderson	No that is not true. These cells are identified by immunofluorescent techniques. One would have to run a complete battery on all smooth muscle cells and myofibroblast to determine the similarities and differences, which has not been done.
William Wagner	In our particular work, since it was brought up, we have run a fairly complete battery. I think the definition is okay because it is not exclusive. Just because a cell has alpha smooth muscle actin does not mean that it is a myofibroblast. Right? I think it's fine.
James Anderson	When I find porous materials in contact skeleton muscle, for example, I do not use the term myofibroblasts, because this could be infiltration of skeletal muscle precursors, which will also contain the alpha smooth muscle cell actin. So this actually brings up another topic. If you are going to identify you have to run the complete battery. And rarely is a complete battery ever run, even genetically.

(d) Final Definition and Voting for "Myofibroblast"

Myofibroblast

> **Primary extracellular matrix (ECM) - secreting cells containing alpha-smooth muscle actin during wound healing and fibrosis and are responsible for the contractility of scar tissue. Myofibroblast progenitors include resident fibroblasts, fibrocytes, pericytes and may also result from epithelial/endothelial to mesenchymal transition. Myofibroblasts sense and modulate ECM stiffness through focal adhesions via integrin binding**

Voting Yes	39
Voting No	9
Abstain	2
Total Votes	50
Number voting Yes or No	48
Percentage Yes Votes	81.25%

The definition achieved Consensus, having more than 75% Yes votes, with absolute number greater than 30.

(e) Further Commentary on the Definition of "Myofibroblast"

In the context that David Williams was given the authority to make minor grammatical alterations, a slightly better wording is as follows; the delegates did not have sufficient time to focus on the grammar and syntax, focusing only on the scientific accuracy. It is this which is confirmed to have consensus:

Myofibroblast

> **Primary extracellular matrix - secreting cells, which contain alpha-smooth muscle actin, that are active during wound healing and fibrosis and are responsible for the contractility of scar tissue by modulation of matrix stiffness through focal adhesions; their progenitors include resident fibroblasts, fibrocytes, pericytes and may also result from epithelial/endothelial to mesenchymal transition**

F Mechanotransduction

(a) Possible Definitions of "Mechanotransduction" Included in Final Program

1. The processes by which cells sense mechanical stimuli and convert them to biochemical signals that elicit specific cellular responses
2. The molecular and cellular processes that are involved with the conversion of mechanical stimuli into biochemical signals[2]

---

[2] Williams DF, Biocompatibility pathways: Biomaterials-induced sterile inflammation, mechanotransduction, and principles of biocompatibility control, *ACS Biomaterials Sci Eng*, 2017, 3(1), 2–35.

(b) James Anderson; Perspectives on "Mechanotransduction" and Suggested Definition

James Anderson	These are four possibilities for the definition of mechanotransduction. Any combination of these could be considered. Only one could be considered. This is what came out of my extensive review of the literature. It provides a little bit more detail, the number four which is the one that David did last year. It provides a little bit more detail in terms of cellular changes.
James Anderson	Number one. "The effect of external physical forces, i.e. tension, compression, shear osmosis leading to changes in cellular migration, proliferation, activation, orientation/elongation, and other responses." The physical forces/stimuli are transmitted to the cell via mechanical receptors such as integrins, ion channels, growth factor receptors, and G protein-coupled receptors. This gives the user an idea of where to look in terms of what type of receptors are involved in their response.
James Anderson	Number two. "The dynamic reciprocity of cell extracellular mechanical interactions mediated by transmembrane integrin receptors that transmit mechanical forces across the cell surface and facilitate the mechanochemical transduction events that control cell function."
James Anderson	Here we got something of a different approach but I think has some valuable information in it. Three. "The processes by which cells sense mechanical stimuli and convert them to biochemical signals that elicit specific cellular responses." Probably the simplest of all definitions. It does not provide the user with additional information as to where to look or what's involved in mechanotransduction.
James Anderson	Then number four, "the molecular and cellular processes that are involved with the conversion of mechanical stimuli into biochemical signals," David's definition.
Andrés García	Okay. Comments from the group?
James Anderson	Oh wait. This can be ... all four can be acceptable. Or any combination of the four. Because this is the one example that we have where we are putting forth several possible definitions for ultimate consideration.

To summarize, the four possible definitions are:

Mechanotransduction

1) The effect of external physical forces, i.e., tension, compression, shear and osmosis, leading to changes in cellular migration, proliferation, activation, orientation/ elongation and other responses. The physical forces/stimuli are transmitted to the cell via mechanoreceptors, such as integrins, ion channels, growth factor receptors, and G-protein coupled receptors

2) The dynamic reciprocity of cell-ECM mechanical interactions mediated by transmembrane integrin receptors that transmit mechanical forces across the cell surface and facilitate mechanochemical transduction events that control cell function and fate

3) The processes by which cells sense mechanical stimuli and convert them to biochemical signals that elicit specific cellular responses

4) The molecular and cellular processes that are involved with the conversion of mechanical stimuli into biochemical signals

(c) Edited Discussion of "Mechanotransduction"

Kristi Anseth	I have liked many of the proposals. I was wondering about something simple, just the ability to alter biological outcomes through mechanical forces.
James Anderson	Where? Where would you?
Andrés García	As a new definition.
Kristi Anseth	A simple definition.
James Anderson	I would agree with you, yes. But there is such a thing as becoming too simple. It does not to provide the reader with a direction, focus, or vision to follow. Remember, I am targeting the future.
Rena Bizios	I like the simplicity aspect. However, it does not give me the important aspect of mechanotransduction. The cellular level. We have to have that word there because that is where mechanotransduction takes place. If we do not have this word, cell or signal or something like that, it is an incomplete definition for me.
James Anderson	In answer to Rena's comment, remember this is a general definition to be used by your specific system. It may or may not necessarily fit. You have to use it as you see fit in the context of what you are working with in terms of biomaterials and what you desire as a biomedical device.
David Williams	I quite like 2, 3, or 4. I think they're fine. Number one I think is difficult, it refers to external physical forces. I am not sure in that context what external is because many of our mechanical forces are internal.
James Anderson	Anything outside the cell.
David Williams	Well I do not think you need it.
James Anderson	It is in previous definitions.
David Williams	I like to be simpler here. I'd go with either 2, 3, or 4. I do not like number one. It goes against the point of having too much mechanistic information in there.
James Anderson	But mechanistic information is where the action is going to be. That is where we are going to target our ultimate therapeutics.
David Williams	That does not have to be in the basic definition.
James Anderson	No but it would be helpful to the user of the definition.

Arthur Coury	A pacemaker may have a piezoelectric sensor inside of it. It receives signals by force transmitted through the body's matrix. It has nothing to do with cells. Is that not mechanical transduction, or mechanotransduction?
Andrés García	Can you briefly restate your comment?
Arthur Coury	Just about every pacemaker senses activity. Some of the activity sensors are piezoelectric transducers inside the pacemaker. They sense movement by changes in the pressure across your matrices. This is nothing to do with cells. Is that mechanotransduction or is it not?
James Anderson	No.
Arthur Coury	Why isn't it, if it is not?
James Anderson	Mechanotransduction targets what is happening in the tissue microenvironment adjacent to implants. It is not meant to discuss medical devices per se and those types. That would fall in another category.
Elizabeth Cosgriff-H	I would agree with David on three and four. I would say two has a couple things that are too narrowly defined. The cell-ECM aspect would not cover some of the work, similarly with integrins. I think three and four are more broadly acceptable.
James Anderson	I have a comment. If you look at the last sentence of one, it provides guidelines to the user as to what may be involved in facilitating this transmembrane signal. I think that these are very important. If you want to go with 2, 3, and 4 you do not provide this important information to the user of the definition. I would say that I . . . yes I can agree with doing away with one, although I think one may be actually the best definition. Because it provides direction to the user in terms of identifying mechanotransduction and what controls it, and what is happening at least at the membrane surface. We do not go into what is happening within the cell itself.
Kristi Anseth	In definitions three and four, was there reason to pick "stimuli" instead of "forces"; would it be better to change it to "mechanical forces"?
James Anderson	I just did not want to be too redundant.
Kristi Anseth	I really like three, especially if it were mechanical forces instead.
David Williams	You can have force, but you can also have strain. These may be strain determined rather than force determined.
Kristi Anseth	I did not know what was meant by "stimuli" so maybe that captures both.
Rena Bizios	Another thing that I would like to ask your opinions is if we can specify that you would be the center of responses which are again survival, contributions to new tissue for the measurement of all

physiological and pathological conditions. Something along those lines to expand the scope of what those cellular responses are pertinent to. They are not random pertinent responses. From my perspective, it is tissue healing around the implants that make me make this suggestion.

Timmie Topoleski   I'm going to go back to what Kristi said and I like the term"force" instead of "stimuli." I don't think you can have strains without force. You need forces to generate strains and deformations.

Timmie Topoleski   There has to be an external force to cause the stimulus. Mechanically speaking, right? The cause of the stimulus could be chemical, it could be from other sources.

David Williams   Yes, but it could be strain - induced because you may have a system where you have for example, flexing of a tubular structure and that is strain induced. Then that converts to force.

Timmie Topoleski   Well no, if you have got a flexing structure, it has to be caused by a force. The flexion has to be caused by some force somewhere, which then produces a strain, which then could put a force on something else sure.

David Williams   The force is somewhere else, not necessary at that point.

Timmie Topoleski   It has to be somewhere right? There's going to be some mechanical force.

Timmie Topoleski   I think even if you have a strain somewhere it is going to cause a force on the cell.

David Williams   I agree.

Andrés García   Can we get a quick show of hands, "force" versus "stimulus"? Who would be in favor of force? And stimulus? Seems like there are more stimuli than forces.

James Anderson   But if you look at the, as I mentioned before, if you look at the second sentence of the first definition, it says the physical force is our stimuli. It links the two. You decide on what you want to use; force or stimuli.

Ruggero Bettini   How about using definition three and adding the second sentence of definition one? The processes by which cells sends mechanical stimuli and convert them to biochemical signals that elicit specific responses. The physical forces or stimuli are transmitted to the cell via mechanoreceptors such as blah, blah, blah, blah, blah.

Rena Bizios   I like that suggestion. The only thing you expanded on these details of the transmission of this stimulus mechanical force, whatever it happens to be, but then you leave that stimulus responses not defined.

Ruggero Bettini   Well, then you are back to definition one, right? If you want to define both then we are back to one.

Rena Bizios	No, you need to specify what the cellular responses are for in this particular context of the mechanotransduction.
Ruggero Bettini	But I would argue that the cellular responses are specific to that obligation. I would not want to prescribe them at the definition stage.
Andrés García	Can we vote on ... I'm going to modify, which one do you guys want me to modify? Three. At this second sentence or not? Raise of hands for yes. No, okay? Since we do not have to change it, we are going to be voting on definition three shown on the screen. Okay are we open?

(d) Final Definition and Voting for "Mechanotransduction"

Mechanotransduction

The processes by which cells sense mechanical stimuli and convert them to biochemical signals that elicit specific cellular responses

Voting Yes	46
Voting No	3
Abstain	0
Total Votes	49
Number voting Yes or No	49
Percentage Yes Votes	93.9%

The definition achieved Consensus, having more than 75% Yes votes, with absolute number greater than 30.

G Blood Compatibility

(a) Possible Definitions of "Blood Compatibility" Included in Final Program

No preliminary definition was provided in the conference program; no definition of the term "blood compatibility" resulted from the 1986 Chester conference and, in fact, the term was deprecated because of the difficulty of understanding the complexity of the subject.

(b) James Anderson; Perspectives on "Blood Compatibility" and Suggested Definition

James Anderson	Okay, now we will move to the next block of definitions. Here we have three in this block. Blood compatibility, thrombogenicity, and complement activation.
James Anderson	Blood compatibility is the "ability of a blood contacting material to resist and/or inhibit the formation of a thrombus or blood clot by inhibition of the intrinsic and/or extrinsic blood coagulation pathways and blood platelet activation."

The suggested definition was, therefore:

Blood Compatibility

The ability of a blood contacting material to resist and/or inhibit the formation of a thrombus or blood clot by inhibition of the intrinsic and/or extrinsic blood coagulation pathways and blood platelet activation

(c) Edited Discussion of "Blood Compatibility"

Editor's Note: As with "inflammation," one discussion took place during Session II, discussed here in Part One. Because of difficulties with this discussion, the conference returned to the subject in the Final Session, discussed in Part Two.

PART ONE: Discussion in Session II

Ruggero Bettini	The definition does not take into consideration the hemolysis.
John Brash	I have a couple comments on blood compatibility. I think that we are being a little soft here by saying "resist" and "inhibit." I would like to be stronger and say to be blood compatible, it should prevent the formation of a thrombus or a blood clot. That's one sentence. The first part should say the "ability to prevent the formation of a thrombus and blood clot." The second part should introduce the same thought into it by saying blood clotting via the extrinsic and intrinsic pathways is not inhibited. Platelets do not adhere to the material and are not activated. That is a lot closer to what I would call blood compatibility than the wording which is used in this definition.
John Brash	The second point is that some of us in this field are trying to develop materials which allow the clotting of thrombus to actually go ahead to a very, very limited extent. Then we design a material so that it will destroy, lyse the clot or thrombus as it forms before it can do major damage. That could be another definition of blood compatibility. You allow it to happen, but the material has properties that will lyse the thrombus as it forms before it can do damage.
Hua Ai	We are talking about blood compatibility, about the material which comes into contact with blood cells and their response, including thrombosis and hemolysis. The key aspects may involve all blood cells, maybe neutrophils and lymphocytes. How about if the material does not generate thrombosis or hemolysis but does some damage or whatever with these kinds of cells. We should include all in the compatibility definition.
Carl Simon	You could adapt the biocompatibility definition and make it a little more general. The ability of a material to perform within an appropriate response in blood in a specific application.
Andrés García	You have to have a little bit more specificity in the definition. Make it really usable and useful to people who are trying to work in the field.

William Wagner	I agree with a lot of the earlier comments. Hemolysis has to be a part of blood compatibility. Complement activation has to be a part of blood compatibility and a relative perspective on what is compatible I think needs to be a part of it. Just as it is for biocompatibility. A Dacron vascular graft for aortic aneurysm repair is adequately blood compatible, but we all know it is modestly thrombogenic. I think if you're talking about coronary vascular grafts and synthetic vascular grafts, we cannot do that. We are not at that level of blood compatibility. It varies in terms of what is compatible. It depends upon the application that you are talking about, just like "biocompatibility" does. I think the definition should reflect somewhat that relative nature of the term.
Arthur Coury	So Cato may remember your former colleague from the University of Connecticut who discovered that with pyrolytic carbon heart valves, platelets adhere so strongly and spread so wide that you can hardly tell that they are there permanently and they inactivate or they passivate that surface. You could have blood compatibility generated by these very strong actions. I really agree with Carl that compatibility is very similar to that in other tissues.
Rena Bizios	I am not convinced that platelets will make the surface blood compatible but that is beside the point. I agree with some of the comments that were made earlier, namely in terms of including the complement activation or other humoral components. But Art mentioned some kind of passivation of a surface. He has been proven many times, I think we can say somehow the surface is considered passivated.
Rena Bizios	There is an addition to complement, some other humeral components, another aspect that was mentioned earlier. What we are covering in these definitions so far is the prevention of the blood clot, or the process which leads to the prevention of the blood clot, but in actual fact we have the other aspect, which is the capability of breaking down that clot once it has formed. There is a separate definition or some part of this definition. A blood compatible material should have not only the ability to prevent the blood clot formation, but capability, when the time comes, to break it down.
Cato Laurencin	Just a small comment from the clinical world. Again, in terms of looking at blood compatibility, when we create grafts for arterial bypass, the first thing that we do is we actually pass blood through the graft, and just from my old cardiac surgery days, we actually have it pre-clot. We actually have it in interact, clot, and then we implant it in the patient. So there's a clotting step that we actually have to make for vascular grafts during the phase before we actually implant them. It is a case of something where you need

	blood compatibility, and you need clotting to take place in order to be able to surgically use it.
Bikramjit Basu	I was wondering that whether we can add that at the last of the definition, and the blood platelet activation under blood flow conditions. That flow is missing in the thrombogenicity. We have mentioned that under the dynamic flow. Here, in the blood compatibility definition, whether we can add this under the blood flow condition.

(d) Final Definition and Voting for "Blood Compatibility"

Blood Compatibility

The ability of a blood contacting material to resist and/or inhibit the formation of a thrombus or blood clot by inhibition of the intrinsic and/or extrinsic blood coagulation pathways and blood platelet activation

Voting Yes	19
Voting No	29
Abstain	0
Total Votes	48
Number voting Yes or No	48
Percentage Yes Votes	39.6%

The definition achieved neither consensus nor provisional consensus.

PART TWO: Discussion in Final Session

Editor's Note: Following the discussions in Session II, several delegates tried to come up with a modified definition that could be discussed again. The following is the preferred option that arose.

"The ability of a blood-contacting biomaterial to (1) avoid the formation of a thrombus by minimal activation of blood coagulation and platelet deposition, (2) promote fibrinolysis, (3) experience minimal activation of the complement system and (4) minimize hemolysis"

David Williams	I agree that is better. I had one comment on that one. In that "ability," does that require all four components? And specifically, for blood compatibility, do you have to promote fibrinolysis? Whoever produced that, I like the idea, but I am not sure that to have blood compatibility it is mandated that you do that.
John Brash	Well, Rena and I put that in there, which was in response to some of the discussion we had yesterday on this. Actually, looking at it now, I would agree that it is not a necessity. It is a nice thing to think about, and I have thought about it. Maybe that's why it is there, but I am not sure that it needs to be in that list.
John Brash	I had two thoughts when I was doing this. One was to beef up some of the words that were used originally. Things like "inhibit."

	I wanted to actually use "prevent." I now see that it has been watered down to "minimal activation" as opposed to "prevention." I guess I am okay with that. And then to include some of the other things, since we had focused mainly on thrombosis yesterday. We said we need to include the complement system and hemolysis. So these are the thoughts. But I would agree to take out number two. If that is offensive or felt not to be necessary.
David Williams	Fine. In other words, it is not mandated. But I think whoever made that comment yesterday you could achieve blood compatibility largely by promoting fibrinolysis. Is that possible?
John Brash	It might be included under one, because it is really intended to be combined with the avoidance of thrombosis.
David Williams	So the suggestion is to take out "promote fibrinolysis," because that may be implied within the option one.
John Brash	Or it could be mentioned in that.
David Williams	Okay, yes. "Avoid the formation of a thrombus by minimal activation of blood coagulation and platelet deposition, and possibly promoting fibrinolysis"?
John Brash	Or "promotion of fibrinolysis."
William Wagner:	Okay, very good. Yes.
Elizabeth Cosgriff-H	I think it was Bill maybe yesterday was talking about that there is a relative need of these aspects in each application. So I think something more, harkening back to the biocompatibility, which is the ability of a blood contacting biomaterial to function in a given application without negative consequence by some combination of these actions. So something that gives that relative aspect to it.
Cato Laurencin	So again with some implants we actually count on a thrombus being formed. You want to form a layer of thrombus on a vascular graft before we implant it.
John Brash	Cato, is that not to seal the prosthesis against leakage as opposed to anything to do with it causing thrombosis?
Cato Laurencin	Yes, one part of it is the sealant.
Arthur Coury	Cato is referring to a device, not a biomaterial.
John Brash	Yes, true.
James Anderson	There is a difference.
Arthur Coury	But isn't that how we define blood compatibility in terms of a device? It is the ability of a material to perform - for the material to allow the device to perform as it should. And to me it is the same thing. Yesterday I mentioned how avidly carbon causes platelets to activate and to spread, and thereby making it a blood compatible surface. But it is not by minimizing platelet adhesion. It is maximizing platelet adhesion, maximizing platelet activation.
James Anderson	I would argue against this; I want to argue against Art.

Cato Laurencin	Well, I think this is a very good point there. There are things that you actually buy to clot. So, you know, the Avitene material, millions of dollars are spent every year on Avitene. We use that when there is a lot of bleeding around and we need a blood clotting biomaterial that we can put in that actually causes it to quickly clot. So again, so that is a biomaterial that we utilized purely for clotting.
William Wagner	I think a couple of things. Fibrinolysis is one mechanism. You could also say nitric oxide generation. You could say, prostacyclin release, you could say a lot of different things that would reduce thrombosis risk. So I favor just taking it out. Then the second point. There is a number of devices that you do want clotting, for example an aneurysm coil. You want that to clot. Hemostatic agents, you want to clot.
James Anderson	It is not a clot, it is a thrombus.
William Wagner	By and large, no. A thrombus would be pathologic, and the clot would be non-pathologic.
William Wagner	So, the other point I would make is that these devices exist, by and large, when you see the term blood compatibility, people do not assess compatibility of hemostatic agents. They assess their ability to do that. So it is an exception. We could maybe change the wording somehow, take knowledge that there are some devices, but by and large, your thrombus implies pathology and complement. I cannot think of any device where you want complement to be activated. And hemolysis? Same thing. I do not know of any device where you want hemolysis to happen.
Laura Poole-Warren	I was just going to put in a vote for Elizabeth's suggestion. I think that something like "the ability of a material to perform in blood contacting applications with appropriate levels of thrombus hemolysis and complement activation" or something like that, might make more sense and the line with biocompatibility as well.
Rena Bizios	We have to use more strong terms, and you have to use active verbs instead of passive verbs. For example, the very experience is a passive verb in my opinion. "Avoid" and "minimize" are active verbs. In addition to the deposition of platelets, platelets by their deposit, they're not going to do anything in my opinion. They have to be activated. That word has to be changed to "platelet activation" for sure.
Rena Bizios	And in addition, the things that Bill mentioned in terms of prostacyclin and nitrogen oxide production, yes, they are all aspects of implementing blood compatibility factors. Let me rephrase that, thrombi formation. Once they are formed, the physiological system brings in fibrinolysis.

Rena Bizios	In my opinion, the blood compatible materials have to include that capability, that particular aspect, and we have to bring to the attention of the people who are going to be using these definitions, not only in the past, but the future.
David Williams	I have to say I have a feeling we are going around in circles here. It is the same circle we went around yesterday morning. I think I mentioned then we could not achieve any agreement in Chester on the same topic and I think for very good reasons, one of which is, of course, blood compatibility has to be seen in the context of the hemodynamics, which is not in this definition at all. And I think whether it is a material or device is a hugely important issue.
John Brash	Yes, I agree with that. Some people believe it is also related to the material itself, which I disagree with.
David Williams	I think we did not achieve consensus yesterday for a good reason, and that is that it is so difficult to define blood compatibility per se by itself. So the question is do we pursue this anymore this afternoon, or do we say within the text that it is roughly the same discussion we had yesterday, and it was not possible to achieve agreement here for very good reasons.
John Brash	Why are we not having agreement? I mean, it seems to come down to the question of including things about materials that promote thrombosis. I can't imagine having that in the definition of blood compatibility, something that promotes thrombus.
David Williams	Yes, I agree John, but I am hearing different ideas around the table. I am worried that we are not going to achieve agreement or consensus however long we go.
William Wagner	Do you do want to assess it in the device as well. We are talking about a biomaterial, so neglecting major flow affects, the thing that they are worried about is platelet deposition and not a single monolayer of spread out platelets but significant platelet deposition leading to a thrombus which would be of significance, complement activation, and hemolysis. Those are the big three that we are worried about.
David Williams	Okay, do you want to put that in a definition?
William Wagner	I think maybe a simplistic definition where yes, we haven't worried about hemostatic agents or aneurysm coils. We haven't worried about embolic agents, things like that, but I think we could address the term that is used all over the place in our literature.
David Williams	There are some issues there, abused.
William Wagner	Exactly. That is why I think it would be useful to have a term that kind of lays out what you should have behind it when you start talking about blood compatibility.
David Williams	Fine, if you think that we can in five minutes produce that definition.
William Wagner	I do not think we can. I mean based on the conversation.

David Williams	Fine. Let's do that then, we will come back and have further discussion.
John Brash	No, let us wordsmith it a little bit.
David Williams	Okay, John wants to wordsmith slightly. Go ahead.
John Brash	I think it is platelet activation, not deposition. Platelet activation, not simple deposition. I would not vote for just deposition.
William Wagner	That is a pretty bland definition.
David Williams	You happy then to take a vote on that?
William Wagner	I would take out fibrinolysis.
John Brash	I wouldn't vote for it then.
Serena Best	Can we get rid of that?
David Williams	Are you saying do we need two activations there?
Rena Bizios	Experience is just a ridiculous word.
David Williams	With a caveat, that's not perfect wording. But I am happy to do some wordsmithing afterwards in view of the time. Could we vote on that? With that caveat, it might change slightly?
Kazunori Kataoka	How do you think of the relation between blood compatibility and non-thrombogenicity.
William Wagner	I would say there is non-thrombogenicity, there is anti-thrombogenicity, and there is thromboresistance. And thromboresistant and non-thrombogenic are subsets of blood compatibility because you could have complement activation or hemolytic activity, even though it is thromboresistant.
Kazunori Kataoka	Yes. I am talking about a graft. So sometimes it is kind of the blood compatible. But if you define blood compatibility like this, then the graft should not be part of blood compatible materials.
William Wagner	Gore-Tex would be okay.
Kazunori Kataoka	It is an activator.
William Wagner	Yes, and that is why we use words like "avoid" and "minimal" because it acknowledges that Gore-Tex and Dacron for that matter are modestly thrombogenic, but it's not of substantial impact - you cannot make a three-millimeter vascular graft out of Gore-Tex, but you can make an eight-millimeter one.
Kazunori Kataoka	Any material cannot survive, for example. Yes, not any materials can be compatible if the blood rate is so strong. So always, in how do you say is contacting with circulating blood it is always an issue of the shear rate and the blood rate. So I am little bit too concerned about this definition.
William Wagner	So there is device biocompatibility and biomaterial blood compatibility. The biomaterial, we seek to isolate just the material contribution independent of the flow, and independent of the status of the blood.
Kazunori Kataoka	So that means that this always a case which maybe the materials or device used in the always under the blood flow.

William Wagner	It depends on the rate of the flow. And yes, there is probably going to be some kind of flow, but it is potentially going to vary greatly.
David Williams	Okay, so John?
John Brash	I am trying to find the intrinsic property of the material itself, at least as far as I know in this exercise, which does not depend on the flow at all. In the device, certainly it does.
David Williams	Okay, at this point, we have a choice of either trying to vote on this, or anybody immediately comes up with an alternative. I think Bill has already declined that.
William Wagner	Well, no just I said my controversial comment that I think fibrinolysis is a subset of techniques. I don't think it rises to the definition of blood compatibility.
John Brash	It is the mirror image of formation, it is formation or destruction. I think that is in a different category from, for example a release of nitric oxide, which is one of the things that you had that pointed out.
David Williams	I think we are going to have to take a vote on this as we have on the screen now.
John Brash	Now number two should probably read "avoids activation of the complement system" as opposed to "experience minimal" or "avoids activation."
William Wagner	Minimizes activation.
Rena Bizios	That is okay, too.
David Williams	I think "minimizes" is better than "avoids," but take out "experience."
Rena Bizios	"Minimize" is fine.
John Brash	Yes, I do not know. If you look at the preamble to the numbers, it says "the ability of a blood contacting biomaterial to…."
David Williams	To minimize.
Rena Bizios	Okay.
David Williams	So after number two, to "minimize activation the complement system,"
David Williams	Okay, that's fine.

(e) Final Definition and Voting for "Blood Compatibility"

Editor's Note: As the above discussion shows, there was much comment on the final wording and syntax, such that the editor was asked to carry out some grammatical adjustments. The following definition arises from this:

Blood Compatibility

The ability of a blood-contacting biomaterial to (1) avoid the formation of a thrombus by minimal activation of platelets and of blood coagulation, (2) minimize activation of the complement system and (3) minimize hemolysis

Voting Yes	29
Voting No	15
Abstain	1
Total Votes	45
Number voting Yes or No	44
Percentage Yes Votes	65.9%

The definition achieved provisional consensus with over 50% Yes votes.

H Thrombogenicity

(a) Possible Definitions of "Thrombogenicity" Included in Final Program

The property of a material which induces and/or promotes the formation of a thrombus; *Definition that achieved consensus in Chester 1986*

(b) James Anderson; Perspectives on "Thrombogenicity" and Suggested Definition

James Anderson	Next, thrombogenicity. The formation of a thrombus and the process is called thrombosis. Through surface activation of the coagulation pathways and platelet activation as well as blood flow, turbulence, or stasis.

(c) Edited Discussion of "Thrombogenicity"

Ruggero Bettini	According to me, this is not the definition of thrombogenicity, it is a definition of thrombogenesis.
James Anderson	The definition of what?
Ruggero Bettini	Thrombogenesis.
James Anderson	Thrombosis and thrombogenesis are the same.
Ruggero Bettini	My comment is that the thrombogenicity should be the tendency or the ability of the material to generate a thrombosis.
Carl Simon	In the form of the word up there, it doesn't align. The description. You are just saying alter the term.
Nicholas Peppas	I tend to agree with Ruggero. Thrombogenesis and thrombogenicity are two totally different words. Thrombogenicity talks about the result of the genesis. Now if all of us in this field are using the two terms the same way that is another story. But it is not correct.
James Anderson	"Resist" and "inhibit" are what it does.
John Brash	Can we consider changing the word at the beginning, as was discussed? Yes, there was discussion about the formation versus the property of the material, thrombogenicity ...

Rena Bizios	Versus thrombogenesis.
John Brash	Versus thrombogenesis.
Carl Simon	Our option was just to change the definition to thrombogenesis.
John Brash	That would work.
Carl Simon	Thrombogenicity is the term.
Laura Poole-Warren	Thrombogenicity, the term could be a tendency of a material in contact with the blood too blah, blah.
Andrés García	The tendency to what?
Laura Poole-Warren	Tendency of a material in contact with the blood.
William Wagner	I did not register my dissatisfaction with the term aside from the Latin correction that we did. You do not have to have surface activation of the coagulation pathway to have platelet deposition onto a surface. You do not have to have turbulence, and stasis is a condition of a medical device, not of a biomaterial.
James Anderson	Exactly. Our target is medical devices, not biomaterials.
William Wagner	In the context of assessment, because you assess thrombogenicity, you can assess thrombogenicity of a material or you can assess it of a device, they are different things.
James Anderson	Regulatory approval requires you to.
William Wagner	This says the tendency of a material, not the tendency of a device.
Andrés García	Can I add slash device? Would that take care of your . . .
William Wagner	You are pointing out the different points of Virchow's triad and I think the point, the part of Virchow's triad that we are interested in is the material inherent thrombogenicity. Of course, if you have stasis, if you have high shear you are going to push the tendency towards more thrombosis. But, in and of itself, the material has an inherent thrombogenicity associated with it. It does not have to involve necessarily high levels of intrinsic cascade, extrinsic cascade, just outright platelet activation on the surface. I think a simpler definition is better. I think what was mentioned before is the "tendency of a material in contact with blood to form a thrombus." Just end it right there.
Andrés García	Bill, we want to also have this as a target for medical devices, not just biomaterials. After all, what are biomaterials being created for? Medical devices. We want to expand this a little bit so that the person reading the definition understands that the biomaterial ultimately is target for a medical device.
William Wagner	Right, but it gets back to the argument about mechanisms. You could say the tendency of a material or device in contact with blood to form a thrombus, and I would be fine with that. You could talk about all of Virchow's triad aspects playing a potential

	role, but the way that it is worded now, it says through this, this, as well as this. It is not necessarily all of them, each one of them can have a more dominant or less dominant role.
Ruggero Bettini	I would comment in saying that when you are dealing with a medical device you look for the tendency of the material constituting the medical device, not the medical device by itself. It is the material that generates the thrombogenicity, not the device.
David Williams	I wholeheartedly agree with Bill, I think we can keep it that simple. I do not like the end of the sentence, but the first part, putting the material and/or medical device, I think that is perfectly satisfactory. This discussion shows why in Chester back in 1996 we could not get consent to any of these definitions, and roughly the same discussion went on. We have to bear in mind in the comment that blood compatibility is controlled by the material characteristics and the hemodynamics. It's very difficult to separate those out if we go into a more complex definition.
Andrés García	I am going to make the executive decision to modify this to and thrombosis, as Bill suggested, and we will take a vote in that.
Andrés García	Let me change that quickly here so we can vote. Please vote. Is it open?

(d) Final Definition and Voting for "Thrombogenicity"

Thrombogenicity

The tendency of a material in contact with blood to form a thrombus

Voting Yes	47
Voting No	1
Abstain	0
Total Votes	48
Number voting Yes or No	48
Percentage Yes Votes	93.9%

The definition achieved Consensus, having more than 75% Yes votes, with absolute number greater than 30.

I Complement Activation

(a) Possible Definitions of "Complement Activation" Included in Final Program

Process in which serum proteins of the complement system are involved in sequential activation by antibody-antigen complexes, cell walls or biomaterial surfaces, that produces effector molecules involved in inflammation, phagocytosis and other biological responses

(b) James Anderson; Perspectives on "Complement Activation" and Suggested Definition

James Anderson	And the last one, complement activation. This should actually be one and two. A cascade of enzymatic reactions that when activated, produce defective molecules involved in implementation, cell adhesion, phagocytosis, and cell lysis. The second definition is a process in which serum proteins of the complement system are involved in sequential activation by antigen antibody ... by antibody antigen complexes, cell walls, or biomaterial surfaces that produce effector molecules involved in inflammation, phagocytosis, and other biological responses.
Rena Bizios	My friendly suggestion is that we need here to specify the cells. There have to be white blood cells. In my limited knowledge of the events, they are the protagonist of the complement activation. Right? Or not?
James Anderson	The inflammation has white blood cells.

(c) Edited Discussion of "Complement Activation"

There was very little constructive discussion about complement activation. On balance the group preferred the first option proposed by the plenary speaker.

(d) Final Definition and Voting for "Complement Activation"

Complement Activation

A cascade of enzymatic reactions that when activated produce effector molecules involved in inflammation, cell adhesion, phagocytosis and cell lysis

Voting Yes	43
Voting No	1
Abstain	4
Total Votes	48
Number voting Yes or No	44
Percentage Yes Votes	97.7%

The definition achieved Consensus, having more than 75% Yes votes, with absolute number greater than 30.

J Macrophage Phenotype

(a) Possible Definitions of "Macrophage Phenotype" Included in Final Program

None was included as the term was not on the original list of terms to be discussed.

(b) James Anderson; Perspectives on "Macrophage Phenotype" and Suggested Definition

James Anderson   This is the last definition. It is "macrophage phenotype": The expression of endocrine, exocrine, paracrine, and membrane functions related to the resolution of inflammation tissue repair and remodeling in response to signals from various stimuli macrophages undergo a reprogramming, leading to the emergence of a spectrum of distinct functional phenotypes in a stimuli dependent continuum ranging in polarization states from pro-inflammatory (classically activated M1 phenotype) to anti-inflammatory (alternatively activated M2 phenotype), what's the rest?

(c) Edited Discussion of "Macrophage Phenotype"

James Anderson   This is included to give a more definitive understanding of the macrophage and what it can do.[3] This was included because of the conflict that results in the literature between people that are either lumpers or splitters. If you are a splitter you talk about M1 versus M2. When in fact it may be a continuum and so it is all lumped into one large continuum. This has led to significant confusion in people trying to determine whether a biomaterial is pro-inflammatory or is anti-inflammatory? This helps to understand the macrophage phenotype. It is what happens when it interacts at a biomaterials surface.

Arthur Coury   Is the word "resolution" the best word? I know it is related to the generation, and if you have chronic inflammation are you resolving the macrophage response?

James Anderson   That's a commonly used term in pathophysiology which in essence says it goes away.

Arthur Coury   But does it always go away?

James Anderson   What?

Arthur Coury   A foreign body giant cell could be there for years.

James Anderson   Of course. I am talking about macrophages.

Arthur Coury   Macrophages are also there with foreign body giant cells throughout.

James Anderson   They may or may not be.

Andrés García   Art, do you have a better word for "resolution"?

James Anderson   I would argue strongly against any other word.

Andrés García   David?

David Williams   I am not sure about another word but I think I see where Art is going here. The second line refers to the resolution of

---

[3] Mantovani A, Biswas SK, Galdiero MR, Sica A, Locati M, Macrophage plasticity and polarization in tissue repair and remodeling, J. Pathol 2013;229:176—85.

inflammation, tissue repair, and remodeling, but then later on we talk of a range of polarization states from pro-inflammatory. If it is pro-inflammatory, that doesn't sound like it is resolving to me, but those are both included.

James Anderson   I missed the point.

Andrés García   That it's the word "resolution" and if you have a pro-inflammatory state is that consistent with a resolution?

James Anderson   No, it's not.

David Williams   When I said there that you have resolution of inflammation, tissue repair, and remodeling, should it be and/or?

James Anderson   That is okay, accepted.

Mário Barbosa   Just two minor points. In the first sentence I think it is perhaps clear, but it could be clearer if we put the macrophage there when you talk about membrane functions, I think it is not cells in general, it is macrophages. In the second sentence maybe "in response to signals from various stimuli, signals from the microenvironment" or "in response to the microenvironment."

James Anderson   No, not necessarily. I understand your first point, but it is obviously assumed that it is the macrophage which is expressing these factors, which are endocrine, exocrine, paracrine, and have the membrane function.

Mário Barbosa   It is implicit.

James Anderson   Yes. In response to your second, for example interleukin-1 is produced by macrophages, but then can be expressed outside the cell and yet come back to the interleukin-1 receptor and interact. That's been described in the literature.

Mário Barbosa   But the sentence, signals from various stimuli is very . . .

James Anderson   Right, and it can be the macrophage itself which is producing the stimuli, releasing it, and then having it react with the same macrophage to change the phenotype.

Xiaobing Fu   It is my opinion that reprogramming and phenotype changes are quite different. Phenotype changes is some gene opens, some gene is closed. Reprogramming is quite different. I don't think it's suitable for this definition.

James Anderson   He is suggesting a change to what?

Xiaobing Fu   Maybe it is possible it is a phenotype change. Reprogramming is not a suitable word here.

James Anderson   What is suitable?

Xiaobing Fu   It is not suitable.

Andrés García   What would you use instead of . . .

Xiaobing Fu   What is suitable, it is "phenotype changes."

Andrés García   Instead of reprogramming.

Xiaobing Fu   Not a reprogramming, it is a phenotype change.

James Anderson	I will buy that, that's fine.
Brendan Harley	Elizabeth and I were just talking about the end also, potentially looking at we have pro-inflammatory but then instead of anti-inflammatory is there ...
Andrés García	Repetitive.
Brendan Harley	Pro wound healing or something that is ...
James Anderson	No, these are classic definitions.
Brendan Harley	I am just, I don't know, I like "constructive."
William Wagner	The term "constructive remodeling" is often used for the anti-inflammatory state in the context of biological scaffolds.
James Anderson	It does not have to be included.
Rena Bizios	Exactly because here we are talking about macrophage phenotype so I think it is okay the way it is.
Andrés García	Any more discussion?
James Anderson	We had that suggestion for the change for reprogramming.
Andrés García	I am going to make that.
James Anderson	In reference to Bill's comment, if one is seriously considering this definition, they will get into the swamp known as the M1-M2 controversy and find out how it has been variously described, or you would argue with the word swamp? Not at all.
Andrés García	The phenotype change, just close the parentheses.
Moderator	Are we ready to vote? Please vote.

(d) Final Definition and Voting for "Macrophage Phenotype"

Macrophage Phenotype

The expression of endocrine, exocrine, paracrine, and membrane functions related to the resolution of inflammation tissue repair and remodeling. In response to signals from various stimuli, macrophages undergo a phenotypic change, leading to the emergence of a spectrum of distinct functional phenotypes in a stimuli-dependent continuum ranging in polarization states from pro-inflammatory (M1 phenotype) to anti-inflammatory (M2 phenotype)

Voting Yes	39
Voting No	10
Abstain	0
Total Votes	49
Number voting Yes or No	49
Percentage Yes Votes	79.6%

The definition achieved Consensus, having more than 75% Yes votes, with absolute number greater than 30.

(e) Further Commentary on the Definition of "Macrophage Phenotype"

In the context that David Williams was given the authority to make minor grammatical alterations, a slightly better wording is suggested; the delegates did not have sufficient time to focus on the grammar. It is this which is confirmed to have consensus.

In particular, the form of this definition is inconsistent with the general rules suggested in an early section of these Proceedings, where definitions of terms related to biomaterials should be consistent with those of the terms in general use. Moreover, definitions should not discuss mechanisms. The term "phenotype," as a noun, is generally held to be "the set of observable characteristics of a cell resulting from the interaction of its genotype with the environment." A better definition of macrophage phenotype would therefore be:

Macrophage Phenotype

The characteristic endocrine, exocrine, paracrine, and membrane functions of macrophages affecting the resolution of inflammation, repair and remodeling; there is a spectrum of distinct functional phenotypes in a stimuli dependent continuum, ranging in polarization states from pro-inflammatory M1 phenotype to anti-inflammatory M2 phenotype

K Other Biocompatibility-Related Terms: No Voting, With or Without Discussion

A number of other terms were scheduled for discussion and voting during Session II but time allowed for only limited discussion and no votes were taken. The definitions proposed by the Plenary Speaker are included here for completeness.

Bioactivity

A phenomenon by which a biomaterial elicits or modulates biological activity

Bioactive Material

A material which has been designed to induce specific biological activity *Definition that achieved consensus in Chester 1986.*

Immunity

Refers to innate immunity (inflammation) and/or adaptive/acquired immunity

Foreign Body Reaction

The cellular reaction of the biomaterial/tissue that is initiated by monocyte adhesion to the adsorbed blood protein layer with subsequent monocyte differentiation to macrophage formation that may fuse to form (multinucleated) giant cells, i.e., foreign body giant cells

Fibrosis

The end-stage of the healing response resulting in a multi-layered collagen (Type III) predominant, relatively avascular fibrous capsule

Endothelialization/Epithelialization

The re-establishment of a normal endothelial lining or a normal epithelial surface, respectively

Carcinogenicity

1) The species-dependent potential of a biomaterial to promote the formation of a tumor, usually a sarcoma, at the site of a biomedical device or biomaterial
2) Ability or tendency to produce cancer
   Note that although tumorigenicity is a better term technically since all cancers involve tumors but not all involve carcinomas, carcinogenicity is the preferred term because of greater common use

Granuloma

The foreign body reaction commonly observed with small particles such as polyethylene wear products or suture materials

Granulation

Reparative connective tissue that consists of new capillaries in an edematous environment of fibroblasts, myofibroblasts, inflammatory cells and cellular debris

Necrosis

A pathway of cell death resulting from environmental perturbations with cell membrane rupture and the uncontrolled release of inflammatory cellular constituents

Apoptosis

A pathway of programmed cell death that avoids cell membrane rupture and the initiation of an inflammatory response

Autophagy

A process by which a cell eats itself by delivery of cytoplasmic materials to lysosomes for degradation

Cytokines

Proteins produced by many cell types (principally activated lymphocytes, macrophages and dendritic cells, but also endothelial, epithelial and connective tissue cells) that mediate and regulate immune and inflammatory reactions

Growth Factors

Proteins that stimulate the activity of genes required for cell growth and cell division and may also mediate cellular migration, differentiation and synthetic activities

Osseointegration

The capability of substrate-adherent osteoblasts to produce bone

Osteoclast

Large multinuclear cell associated with absorption and removal of bone

Osteoinduction

Action or process of stimulating osteogenesis

Osteoconduction

Process of passively allowing bone to grow and remodel over a surface

Inflammasome

1) A cytosolic multiprotein complex formed by extracellular stimuli interacting with cell membrane receptors that results in the activation of an enzyme (caspase-1) leading to the production of Interleukin-1, a mediator of acute inflammation
2) A multiprotein intracellular complex that detects pathogenic microorganisms and sterile stressors and that activates the highly pro-inflammatory cytokines IL-1b and IL-18
3) A multiprotein cytoplasmic complex which activates one or more caspases, leading to the processing and secretion of pro-inflammatory cytokines

Phagocytosis

The process of uptake or engulfment of small particle, i.e., bacteria, wear particles, microcapsules and nanobiomaterials, by blood white cells, macrophages and other cell types

Neuronal Inflammation/Neuroinflammation

The activation of microglia, which are the resident immune cells of the brain; the cellular microenvironment, which includes not only microglia, but also astrocytes, oligodendrocytes and peripherally derived innate and adaptive immune cells; and the temporal correlation between different activation states of cells (phenotypes)

Hyperplasia

The increase in the number of cells in an organ or tissue in response to a stimulus

Hypertrophy

The increase in the size of cells in an organ or issue in response to a stimulus that increases production of cellular proteins

Immunomodulation

The ability of a biomaterial to modulate the innate and/or adaptive/acquired foreign body reaction and/or healing responses by enhancing or suppressing normal immune cellular responses.

Dendritic Cells

Immune cells resident in various tissues that are antigen-presenting cells for initiating T-lymphocyte responses.

Adhesive Molecules

Molecules such as fibronectin and laminin that permit the attachment to, and movement of, cells within the extracellular matrix (ECM)

Cell Receptor

Cell membrane and cytosol components capable of recognizing and sensing a wide variety of stimuli which lead to specific activation pathways that are dependent on specific stimulus-receptor interactions. See DAMPs and PAMPs

Remodeling

The constant process of ECM and fibrous capsule collagen degradation and synthesis initiated and controlled by chemical, physical, mechanical and other properties of the biomaterial in the in vivo environment.

Remodeling

The process of maturation and reorganization of connective tissue and ECM components influenced by the balance between synthesis and degradation of ECM components

DAMPs

Damage-associated molecular pattern molecules (DAMPs) are endogenous molecules, i.e., cytokines, chemokines, alarmins, etc., that are constitutively expressed and released upon tissue damage, resulting in activation and exacerbation of non-infectious inflammatory responses

PAMPs

Pathogen-associated molecular pattern molecules (PAMPs) are derived from microorganisms and recognized by pattern recognition receptor (PRR)-bearing cells of the innate immune system as well as epithelial cells

Chemokines

A family of small (8 to 10 kD) proteins that act primarily as chemoattractants for specific types of leukocytes

Cell-Surface Receptors

Transmembrane proteins with extracellular domains bind soluble secreted ligands leading to signaling with formation, modification or activation of intermediates by a variety of pathways and, ultimately, the generation of active transcription factors that alter gene expression

Myofibroblasts

Primary extracellular matrix (ECM) - secreting cells containing alpha-smooth muscle actin during wound healing and fibrosis and are responsible for the contractility of scar tissue. Myofibroblast progenitors include resident fibroblasts, fibrocytes, pericytes and may also result from epithelial/endothelial to mesenchymal transition. Myofibroblasts sense and modulate ECM stiffness through focal adhesions via integrin binding

Pseudotumor

A focal enlargement of tissue, with or without an associated biomaterial

Plasticity/Polarization

The capability of cells, in particular macrophages and fibroblasts, to modulate their phenotype and characteristic function over the time course of inflammation, foreign body response, wound healing and remodeling

Extracellular Matrix

The composite material (ECM) in and between cells with both structural and regulatory function. ECM is composed of collagens, fibronectin, elastin, fibrillins, enzymes, proteoglycans, glycosaminoglycans and others

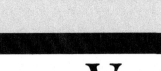

V

Biodegradation phenomena

Discussed in Session I, Session V, and Final General Session

Session I Plenary Presentation: *David Williams*
Session I Moderato: *Kai Zhang*
Session I Reporter: *Carl Simon*
Session V Plenary Presentation: *Nicholas Peppas*
Session V Moderator: *Kazunori Kataoka*
Session V Reporter: *Maria J. Vicent*
Final Session Moderator: *David Williams*
Final Session Reporters: *Carl Simon, Helen Lu, Serena Best*

A Biodegradation

(a) Possible Definitions of "Biodegradation" Included in Final Program

Breakdown of a material mediated by a biological system. *This is a refined version of the 1986 definition (The gradual breakdown of a material mediated by specific biological activity) that eliminates reference to "gradual" and "specific"*

(b) David Williams; Perspectives on "Biodegradation" and Suggested Definition

David Williams	Now one of the terms or group of terms we will discuss I think quite extensively over the next two days concerns biodegradation. There are many different definitions of biodegradation because it isn't only concerned with biomaterials and medical applications. There are many other situations in which "biodegradation" is used and rightly so. In environmental science, for example, if you look at the OEC definition of biodegradation, it says "the process by which organic substances are decomposed by microorganisms, mainly aerobic bacteria into simpler substances such as carbon dioxide, water, and ammonia."
David Williams	That may be a very generic general definition, but I don't think that is good enough for us in biomaterials science. I think we have

to be putting some more detail into the context of biomaterials applications.

David Williams   So I give you two options. The first one actually achieved provisional consensus back in Chester in 1986. "Gradual breakdown of a material mediated by specific biological activity." We may wish to look at a refined, slightly shorter version of that, which I give as, "breakdown of material mediated by a biological system," in which we have removed the emphasis on gradual, because I do not know what gradual really means, and have removed the emphasis on "specific." We may want to look at that.

(c) Edited Discussion of "Biodegradation"

Nicholas Peppas   So David, my question is if the polymer or polymers degrade by hydrolysis while they are in the body, is that biodegradation, is it included or not? Because it appears that you say there has to be a biological reason for the degradation. What about hydrolysis?

David Williams   Nicholas that is a very good point. My "specific biological activity" may be a problem. If it is activity within the biological environment, I believe it is included, but if hydrolysis is purely water and not affected by any other species, which I think is what you are suggesting, is there any reason to exclude that if it is degrading in the biological environment?

Nicholas Peppas   Well I would like the people who did this engineering project to tell me if the scaffold is degraded because of a biological activity or simply because of hydrolysis of PLGA, how is it degraded?

Peter Ma   And I also have that question. It is not just an activity but also could be something in the biological environment, so water actually could be one of the environmental factors. Because biological systems have large amount of water and so I think as you have redefined it as biological activity, so that the environment includes the water.

Maria J. Vicent   I just wanted to comment to compliment the biodegradation definition, because maybe instead of "environment," I think if we just add it is the "biological system" or "physiological activity," or "physiological condition," "biological condition," so we include everything, we can include "pathological situation" and also the environmental hydrolysis or even reductive environment of a cell for example.

Maria J. Vicent   And coming back to "biodegradable polymer," we are saying naturally occurring active species, instead of that saying like "action of the environment" or the "biological condition," instead of being active.

David Williams   Yes.

Maria J. Vicent	I would follow on from Nicholas and the suggestions going to activity…instead of activity going to condition, physiological condition or biological condition so or instead of environment so we will include either activity or also the physiological media and the environment.
David Williams	Are you suggesting we should name those other conditions or just have an alternative word to include them?
Maria J. Vicent	An alternative word to "environment" or "activity."
David Williams	So you are talking about the last option, "breakdown of a material mediated by." instead of "a biological system" you are talking about mediated…
Maria J. Vicent	By a physiological condition. Or biological condition. So that is why we leave it broader to include hydrolysis, reduction environments and so on.
David Williams	Okay, carry on.
James Anderson	I would like to make several comments for your consideration.
James Anderson	First of all, materials do not degrade by water. They degrade by acid. There are three known mechanisms for virtually all of the so-called biomaterials. Acid, reactive oxygen intermediates, and enzymes. And, it is now known that so-called biodegradable polymers may degrade through a combination of any of these. That is well established, and it is actually known clinically.
James Anderson	The second comment I wish to make is that it is possible for materials to undergo so-called surface degradation. The key here is that there is no change in the intended properties of the material for the function when it is in a medical device. I offer you two examples. The first is titanium. Titanium, when implanted, really has a surface, ultimately has a surface of titanium oxide. So, you have changed, in a sense, from a hydrophobic to a hydrophilic material, which certainly has an impact on the interaction with a biological surface.
James Anderson	The second, David - and you know this very well - is polypropylene. Polypropylene may undergo a surface oxidation through the interaction with a reactive oxygen intermediate coming from the cellular microenvironment at the surface. This again, converts a hydrophobic material to a hydrophilic material without having a significant change in the intended properties of the material for its application.
James Anderson	These concepts are subtle, but if you are going to discuss biodegradation, I believe you should consider these possibilities where known mechanisms at the surface of a biomaterial certainly can change its surface properties, but not necessarily its intended,

	or its bulk properties, which may ultimately control the application.
Brendan Harley	I just wanted to add two things. One, about biomaterial, but also I think on the degradation side of things. I agree that there are some questions about how we might define biodegradation and so I was just thinking about . . . There's lots of things that could be biodegradable, meaning they degrade in a biological environment. The question is maybe the mechanism of action and that things that would be processes of biodegradation versus just general degradation. I don't know whether we would think about the definition you have would be an action by a biological environment to drive that process that is more specific, versus just general degradation that could be hydrolysis or other properties as well. I just want to offer that as different thought.
David Williams	Thank you, Brendan. I think that's very helpful. The only issue I have with your first comment is that we end up with a definition which gets into mechanisms. That's what I've tried to say; that's a problem we always have, especially as we don't know all the mechanisms at this point. If we are very specific to, for example, one or two mechanisms, then we become self-limiting. But, I take the point, Brendan.
Elizabeth Cosgriff-H	Regarding the biodegradation, I agree with many of the points raised. I think, in terms of differentiating biodegradation that we are referring to in the body from other biodegradable polymers in the materials, for example, composting that has become very popular as biodegradable materials, I think we need a little bit of wordsmithing on what the biological system is to imply that it is biomedical in target.
Elizabeth Cosgriff-H	Second, in terms of that breakdown, I think it is important for a degradation definition to include a chemical change to differentiate from erosion behavior. Because you have the bioresorption, differentiation of degradation from erosion is important.
James Anderson	I would like to make a comment back on the biodegradation. I may have missed it, but I did not see the term bioerosion.
David Williams	Correct.
James Anderson	Let me remind you, that there are several polymer systems, one of which we have studied, which was polyethylene carbonate, which bioerodes from the surface with a decrease in the mass of the implant, but no change in the molecular weight. That is a unique characteristic; one that's not been fully exploited in the biomaterials area. I would like you to provide, and I don't have a good answer for you at this time, but perhaps later we can, I would like you to

	include bioerosion as a term with a relatively decent definition. Because it certainly is unique when compared to the global term biodegradation.
David Williams	Thank you, Jim. I had assumed, I think correctly, that Nick was going to include bioerosion in terms of drug and gene delivery systems, because that is when it is most relevant. I think you will address that, Nick.
Timmie Topoleski	David, I had a question about the biodegradation and the intention of the definition. You use the word, "breakdown." In the discussion, listening to Jim and Elizabeth speaking of whether it's intentional or not intentional, is the intention of this definition to define loss of function of a biomaterial, because there are some biomaterials that only function when they physically or mechanically break down, and others that lose their function when they degrade. So, if it is to define it as loss of function, maybe replace the word "breakdown" by "loss of function," and that would encompass a larger number of materials.
David Williams	Good point. I deliberately did not include reference to functionality in this definition. I was using the word "breakdown" as part of the general concept of what degradation means. Breakdown can mean a physical, morphological, functional change. My problem is how to change "breakdown" into anything which is equivalent without getting too cumbersome. I agree with what you say, but it is not simple for a biomaterial may not be functional until it has broken down, or may lose functionality once it has broken down. It is very difficult to incorporate that into one definition. That goes back to the point of defining it, and then qualify it in the application.

(d) Final Definition and Voting

Biodegradation

Breakdown of a material mediated within a biological system

Voting Yes	45
Voting No	5
Abstain	0
Total Votes	50
Number voting Yes or No	50
Percentage Yes Votes	90%

The definition achieved Consensus, having more than 75% Yes votes, with absolute number greater than 30.

B Biodegradable Polymer

(a) Possible Definitions of "Biodegradable Polymer" Included in Final Program

1. A polymer which degrades as a result of the action of naturally occurring active species
2. A polymer which degrades as a result of the action of naturally occurring active species where the rate of degradation takes place in a specified time period comparable to existing natural processes

(b) David Williams; Perspectives on "Biodegradable Polymer" and Suggested Definition

David Williams	That leads us then to a "biodegradable polymer." And this is important in many areas of the technology of biomaterials. Our difficulty is that all polymers will interact with a physiological environment to some extent. Essentially biodegradable and biostable polymers provides a very difficult challenge. So my first suggestion for biodegradable polymer is "a polymer that degrades as a result of the action of naturally occurring active species." I've seen several people trying to put that into context of actually what we mean in terms of rate of degradation. So it could be as given in the second possibility where the rate of degradation takes place in a specified time period comparable to existing natural processes. I find it hard to get my mind around exactly what that means but I see it quite often in definitions. So it's either a fairly simple definition, or we can discuss and add that context to it.
David Williams	We then have to look at biostability. Many people in the room refer to biodegradable polymers used in tissue engineering or hopefully biostable polymers used in long-term implantable devices. Art Coury in front of me has worked for a long time in biostable polyurethanes. So what are we meaning by that? Let us note that this is a relative term, since all materials undergo some change over time in biological environments, however small that might be. I think that biostability refers to situations where there are no clinical consequences associated with any change. So my suggestion is, "biostability is the condition in which a material resists chemical and/or structure changes within a biological environment that have clinical consequences," or some variation on that.

Editor's Note: While there are several references to biodegradable polymers in several sessions, in neither Session I nor Session VI, which referenced biodegradable polymers in general and in the context of drug delivery systems, did the discussions lead to any position on a definition and no votes were taken.

C Biodegradable Metal

(a) Possible Definitions of "Biodegradable Metal" Included in Final Program

No definition of "biodegradable metal" was included in the conference program since this was not on the original agenda. However, during Session I, it was agreed that the term could be discussed during the last session if time permitted. Frank Witte produced the following definition in advance of that session:

A pure metal, metal alloy, or composite which is intended to degrade in vivo based on the composition of its biological environment

(b) Edited Discussion of "Biodegradable Metal"

Frank Witte	Yes, thank you David. If you are looking at the list of definitions you have currently proposed there are permanent polymers for implants and biodegradable polymers. These latter polymers should only be there temporarily, to support healing and function. We also have metals, or metallic biomaterials, but we do not have a term for metals that are intended only to be there temporarily, to form a temporary implant material. In the biodegradable metal field, which has been there for more than eighteen years now, implants are already on the market, such as stents and screws, but we do not have a term for the biomaterial.
Frank Witte	In the biodegradable metal community, we were thinking how to form a phrase to basically describe the biomaterial, and this is our proposal "a pure metal, or metal alloy, or composite which is intended to degrade in vivo based on the composition of its biological environment."
David Williams	Thank you Frank. I think we need to take this definition and divide it into two parts for discussion. And the first is, "a pure metal, metal alloy or composite." In this context you cannot have an alloy which is not metallic, so you do not need the second metal there. I'm speaking as a metallurgist.
Frank Witte	Correct, but there are some people trying to apply a pure magnesium and then there are others working on metal alloys. And then there is always a debate, if they are talking about the same. It is true, if you are just talking very generally about metals, it comprises all of this, that is true. In this case, we could take the other terms out.
David Williams	I think we have to take that second "metal" out, and I am not sure what you mean by composite.
Frank Witte	Well a composite compromises a metal part and a non-metallic part.
David Williams	I assumed you would say that, and the metal matrix composite is the only one I know, but it is not obvious because I think, in a

moment we may say we want to define a "biocomposite." And for that, we need to discuss exactly what a composite is.

David Williams   A composite is not just a mixture. And there has to be some very specific parts of that. So I would suggest to be rigorous on that one, I would say "a pure metal, alloy, or matrix metal composite."

David Williams   Right, well let us get to the second part. I think "intended to degrade in vivo" is fairly clear. We do need to discuss this, but "based on the composition of its biological environment" is unclear.

Frank Witte   The point is that we want to distinguish it from permanent implant materials like titanium and cobalt chromium and stainless steel, especially stainless steel, which under certain conditions basically could corrode, which is not intended. It is not designed to degrade in vivo. So this is the difference here. And based on the composition of its biological environment means that the design of the metal alloy or metal matrix composite should be designed in the way that the biological environment is capable to degrade this biodegradable metal.

David Williams   Okay I think we have to discuss that.

Rena Bizios   Then we are willing to substitute its biological environment, because that is now connected to the metal, metal alloy. To the surrounding biological environment.

James Anderson   Yes, I do not think "based on the composition of its biological environment" really adds anything to the definition. It is implied under the word intention. And it is all encompassing.

David Williams   Thank you Jim.

Iulian Antoniac   This definition is missing the purpose of this biodegradable metal. In order to repair or regenerate the damaged tissue. Because, it is not used just to be degraded, without any purpose.

David Williams   Iulian, what was the phrase you say? What was the phrase you wanted to introduce?

Iulian Antoniac   In order to repair or regenerate the damaged tissue. Because for this reason you use these biodegradable metals.

David Williams   That does not include a biodegradable stent.

James Anderson   Yes, this is what I just wanted to say. We just have to be careful about this. It may be just there, not to repair or regenerate tissue, it just can be a temporary auxiliary device, something to hold something together for some period of time or whatever. I think we also have to distinguish between the definition of the metal or the material itself or the device. The material itself I think is not intended to repair tissue.

Rui Reis	David, I am also a metallurgist, but I think we'll have to put back the alloy, because there are polymer alloys. Polymer alloys and special kinds of blends.
David Williams	No.
Rui Reis	Yes, there are.
David Williams	I think that is a total abuse of the word alloy, to add in the word polymer. You have polymer composites and blends, but we do not need "alloys" for polymer systems.
Rui Reis	It's a blend with a controlled interface. They put a dispersed phase to control the interface. So it's a special kind of a polymer blend, it's called a polymer alloy.
David Williams	I will take some other comments, but I personally cannot agree with that one.
Arthur Coury	There is a product called Norel, which is an alloy, and it's been called that for thirty, for forty years, involving styrene and polyphenylene oxide. It is one polymer dissolved in another, it has been accepted in the field. Even though you are a metallurgist, there are polymer alloys.
David Williams	Anybody like to answer that? That may be a commercial description.
David Williams	I think that confuses our definition, but I am willing to take other comments.
Yunbing Wang	I think this is great to add this definition, but what I want to ponder is for polymer, normally, we call it biodegradable polymer or bioresorbable polymer. For metal, normally, we call the biodegradable metal. So, I know. A lot of people also call the biodegradable metal, but at least, I worked in industry for more than 10 years. In industry, normally, we call biodegradable. For metal, when we talked about metal. So, I support to use the term biodegradable. I think it is now it can be unified in the field of biomaterials.
Kai Zhang	Yes, actually, there was a paper published which is discussing the biodegradable, erodible, dissolvable metal. So, I think biodegradable metal, first, I think it is a good word, and also, for the definition, but why do we need the words after "in vivo"? Why don't we just say "a pure metal, alloy, metal matrix compartment, which is intended to degrade in vivo." Why do you care about the rest?
David Williams	That was Jim's suggestion, I think. We'll perhaps come back to that. Bill?
William Wagner	Yeah, I agree with that last suggestion. Cut it after "in vivo." With respect to biodegradable, we have done two special issues on biodegradable metals in our journal. There are conferences on

	biodegradable metals. We are finishing the tenth year of an engineering research center on biodegradable metals. So the term is very well used in the biomaterials literature, I would say.
Peter Ma	I was thinking that is fine for repair or regenerate tissue, but is there a function that you intended to do before it degrades. I think that will be potentially for regeneration, but it could be for other purposes.
Frank Witte	If you look at the definition of biodegradable polymer, there is no functional aspect in the definition of biodegradable polymer because it basically is defining the material itself. So the material itself can be used in different, or for different functions, right? But I think I would not include the function in a definition which should be very broad. That's my idea.
Peter Ma	What I am trying to say is that we should not define one function. But after that, the intended function, then degrade it. Not just desired to degrade.
Frank Witte	The concept is that it is designed to degrade. This is the difference. This metal is designed to degrade in vivo. There are other metals that should last forever.
Peter Ma	I understand that. You need the material to degrade, but the intention is how to function, then degrade after fulfilling that the intended function.
Frank Witte	No. It can fulfill the function while it is degrading. So we should be very careful here. However, there are cases where you do not want to have degradation while it has a function, and then it can degrade. But sometimes it can degrade while it has a function. So there is a huge variety on this and if we try to tackle it in this definition, here, we just need get vague in this part.
David Williams	I tend to agree with that.
Hua Ai	I just have a little problem with "intended." I think biodegradable is a property of the metal no matter if you intend or not. If you just intend, but in reality, it is not.
David Williams	I understand that. I think that is inherent in the fact that all materials, whether they are metal or polymers, are going to degrade to some extent in the body. Even the most corrosion resistant metal, titanium, for example, is to some extent degrading as titanium ions are released. This is specifically designed with this composition to degrade or corrode. That is why I think "intended" is there. And that excludes, then, any other alloy, which is by nature, going to corrode a little bit.
Joachim Kohn	I suggest that we follow exactly the definition of biodegradable polymer, and simply replace polymer with pure metal, alloy, or metal matrix composite. So the two definitions are identical because they just apply to different types of materials. But I think

	the intent of Frank is to have a definition that mirrors the one of the biodegradable polymer.
Frank Witte	Well, exactly. To be similar. I mean we try to improve, actually.
Joachim Kohn	No, that is not part of the definition. From a purely material science perspective, you are designing a material that is intended to degrade in a biological system-
Frank Witte	Correct.
Joachim Kohn	Which is very similar to the definition of the biodegradable polymer. So if we could get back to the biodegradable polymer, and then basically just replace polymer with metal alloy or metal matrix composite, I think we have done this field a great service, because the two definitions should mirror each other because the intent of the materials mirror each other.
Frank Witte	Correct.
David Williams	Thank you, Joachim. I would like to see by a show of hands if people agree with that concept that we should produce a definition here which is analogous for that of biodegradable polymer, and then we will come back to biodegradable polymer later on. Does anybody disagree with that?
David Williams	I think we will come back to that.
Mário Barbosa	I think if you want to go beyond the additional concept of corrosion in vivo, I think we have to put something related to the function that material is going to perform. And if we go back to the definition of bioactive material, we say here that it induces a specific biological function for activity. So I wonder whether instead of the previous definition or part of definition, we could include this purpose.
David Williams	I am not sure. I like the idea of having analogous definition for biodegradable polymer metal, which does not refer to function. Because it could be very many functions. I saw one more over here.
David Williams	I just want to come back to this question of the polymer alloy. I think Rui just left the room at the moment, so I do not want to say it when he is not here, but I have no choice.
David Williams	The title, the word we're defining, is biodegradable metal. It is, therefore, implicit we talk about metallic materials. And that is why I do not think there is any confusion by putting alloy without any reference to a so-called "polymer alloy." I'll explain that to Rui later.
David Williams	Okay. I think I have got agreement here that when we come to biodegradable polymer, we will try to make sure that "biodegradable metal" follows exactly the format with that at the beginning. Is it that agreed we'll do that?

David Williams	I have now found the definition we considered yesterday for "biodegradable polymer," although we did not vote on it. I have to say that I think it's impossible for us to have exactly the same structure for "biodegradable polymer" as with "biodegradable metal." A polymer, as you see in the red towards the top was suggested to be "A polymer which degrades as a result of the action of naturally clearing active species." Maybe with the rest of it. But that is very specific for biodegradable polymer. We are not seeing that with metal.
David Williams	So it was a nice idea to have them in the same structure, but I actually don't think we can. Is that reasonably understood? So we'll go back and have a vote on biodegradable metal.
David Williams	Okay. This is where we got to. We had taken off in that definition … We had taken off in that definition the last part of the phrase. I think most people seem to be happy with keeping it this simple. Frank, you are okay with that?
Frank Witte	That is okay.

(c) Final Definition and Voting

Biodegradable Metal

A pure metal, alloy, or metal matrix composite that is intended to degrade in vivo

Voting Yes	37
Voting No	9
Abstain	0
Total Votes	46
Number voting Yes or No	46
Percentage Yes Votes	80.4%

The definition achieved Consensus, having more than 75% Yes votes, with absolute number greater than 30.

VI

Regenerative medicine

Discussed in Session III and Final General Session

Session III Plenary Presentation: *William Wagner*
Session III Moderato: *Cato Laurencin*
Session III Reporter: *Helen Lu*
Final Session Moderator: *David Williams*
Final Session Reporters: *Carl Simon, Helen Lu, Serena Best*

A Regeneration

(a) Possible Definitions of "Regeneration" Included in Final Program

1. Synthesis of new, natural tissue at the site of a tissue (one cell type) or organ (more than one cell type) which either has been lost due to injury or has failed due to a chronic injury
2. The reactivation of development in later life to restore missing tissues
3. The restoration or new growth by an organism of tissues that have been lost

(b) William Wagner; Perspectives on "Regeneration" and Suggested Definition

William Wagner	Let us move to this concept of regeneration. We have three definitions here, the first; "synthesis of new, natural tissue at the site of a tissue, meaning one cell type or organ meaning multiple cell types, which either has been lost due to injury or has failed due to chronic injury." That is from David Williams' Dictionary of Biomaterial in 1999. Two, "The reactivation of development in later life to restore missing tissues" and similar to number three, "The restoration of new growth by an organism of tissues that have been lost."
William Wagner	I am going to open this up for discussion. I would point out that function is not explicitly been addressed here and that may be something that we want to talk about, whether function is important in defining whether or not something is regenerated or not.

Regeneration

1. Synthesis of new, natural tissue at the site of a tissue (one cell type) or organ (more than one cell type) which either has been lost due to injury or has failed due to a chronic injury; *Williams Dictionary of Biomaterials, 1999*
2. The reactivation of development in later life to restore missing tissues
3. The restoration or new growth by an organism of tissues that have been lost

(c) *Edited Discussion of "Regeneration"*

Cato Laurencin	Any comments, questions? . . . I am going to raise a little bit of an elephant in the room. Should we use the term "functional" and should functional be part of it?
Rena Bizios	In the first definition from tissue it's not only in one cell type arrangement every tissue has more than one cell type so that it needs a little bit more of the vision. Direct division of development in later life is a little bit too broad and too risky in my opinion. But it is not missing tissues; we can combine perhaps some of these concepts of the tissue in the organ on the second one. That is my two reactions, and as far as functional means, I agree with you it should be part of a definition, it has to be functional.
David Williams	Thank you Cato, I am not particularly wedded to the first one, I wrote that nearly 20 years ago. I think it is quite good. The problem I have with number two, it says "restore missing tissues" but tissues don't have to be missing for you to regenerate, especially taking in account your functional concept and I think function is very important to put in there. Again, in number three, the tissues do not necessarily have to be lost, but are no longer functional.
James Anderson	What is the difference between restoration and new growth? In number three.
William Wagner	Yes I think there is an argument to be made that it is redundant. You could have something where there is, for instance, a wholesale new growth as opposed to repopulation or remodeling, or functional remodeling within the tissue, but it's fair enough. I think these three, I myself am not so satisfied with any of them.
James Anderson	I think "new growth" is sufficient.
Kai Zhang	I just want to differentiate regeneration from repair and I do think repair need to be included here as well. In this section it does not say the word, because we are talking about regeneration; it is always associated with repair but I want to see a difference there.
Brendan Harley	So a couple things consensus wise. I think we have got number three, I think that Jim Anderson's point about the fact that restoration or new growth is fine. you don't have restoration there. In terms of tissue and Rena's comment about one cell type, it

actually officially has multiple cell types and probably just taking out the phrase "one cell type" is there.

Kai Zhang	Differentiate regeneration from repair, in my opinion they are different.
Cato Laurencin	So I agree in terms of regeneration, I think it should be restoration of function and you can talk about whether it is through synthesis of new tissue or remodeling process. But repair to me is always scar tissue formation, closing but not necessarily functional. The whole point of regeneration is we do not have to follow a developmental process; sometimes it does and sometimes it doesn't, but the end product is replacement with functional tissue with something that was damaged or lost.
Joachim Kohn	Thank you very much, I think the question about repair is really important because repair is nothing but a different mechanism of regeneration. I think the repair is included in regeneration, but it should be made explicit. Think about muscles, you can regenerate the muscles you have lost as you age. It means you take the weakened muscles and you regenerate new one, you add more tissue mass into it. You could also think about repairing the structure deficit and I really think you should not rush here, you should think about how to combine repair and regeneration and reactivation, restoration because its crucial to the definition really in the fine tuning of the meaning of restoration, repair and regeneration.
Hua Ai	I have a comment on Jim's question, talking about the difference between the restoration and the new growth. Restoration can be considered for example you have artificial blood and it's ready and put into the human being this is restoration and if it's a broken nerve and a tube was there and the new growth of new nerves it is considered new growth. I think maybe that's the difference.
William Wagner	So I'm trying to synthesize some of the comments here. Functional restoration of tissue by an organism, what else?
Cato Laurencin	Yes I think it's fine and then under number three take one out, restoration or leaving new growth.
Xiaobing Fu	It is my opinion if you use force, I am sorry.
Cato Laurencin	Taking out one cell type after number one. I am sorry, go ahead.
Xiaobing Fu	If you use force definitely you'll shoot it, use a structural and a functional restoration because that is recovery so it cannot define the regeneration.
William Wagner	There are some studies going on comparing the newt and the lizard. Whereas the newt when it loses its arm, regenerates an identical and functional arm, the lizard regenerates a functional tail but when you look at the detailed structure it is different. So is the lizard regenerating its tail? I think most people would say yes its

	regenerating its tail even though the function is not exactly reproduced. And with the liver as well, the regenerated liver tissue may not have the exact same original structure but the function is what we generally care about.
Cato Laurencin	While I think function is important, and we have done work where we can actually regenerate arms in salamanders that are not functional, but I think it is something cool to regenerate. Regenerate third arms on animals, so I agree, I think having it as part of it as an important component.
Brendan Harley	Point in clarification. In terms of functional restoration of tissues, the organism part, does that have to be in there? I suppose it needs an active component from wherever it's implanted into but is that superfluous to the definition?
Cato Laurencin	I can see cases where there may be functional restoration, where you destroyed or made something that is working, like a beating heart, but now you are putting out what's outside. Yes?
Cato Laurencin	All right, David?
David Williams	I am wondering does that take into account the treatment of congenital conditions because you are not restoring something, nothings has actually been lost.
Cato Laurencin	Good point, the question is whether it should be, may include functional restoration of a tissue as not something that is definite but something that may be occurring, may be important. Other comments?
Arthur Coury	If we change the word "by an organism" to "in an organism" I mean you might be restoring function by electrical stimulation for example and it might change the tissue. It may be the cause rather than the organism being the cause, what do you think?
Williams Wagner	Not so compelling enough to change it in my opinion. I think it is still the organism if you stimulate it, it is still the organism that is doing it. It doesn't exclude external input.
William Wagner	What about if in this first definition we took out "natural" and we put in "functional?"
William Wagner	We are only talking about regeneration, we have regenerative medicine next to talk about but just the regeneration here.
Cato Laurencin	The different word, different term but you can definitely have an important term in the next point.
William Wagner	Maybe we can knock two of these out.
Cato Laurencin	So if there is a feeling that we have actually put "functional" now in number one so I would suspect that we could take others away and be pretty OK.
Rena Bizios	I think that we can incorporate some of this aspect in the first definition because it is a little bit of redundant after we see the

	injury. Perhaps we can play with words and bring in all aspects of injury but then we can bring in either age which then brings it later in life, or disease because all of these things are part of that.
Cato Laurencin	One or two more we will see if we have a preliminary consensus.
Kristi Anseth	Building on some of the ideas of age and in biology they would normally think every generation is being not just restoration but renewal and growth so if we wanted to, we could say "functional restoration, renewal or growth of tissue by an organism" and that would cover aging, it would cover injury, it would cover going from birth to adult.
Cato Laurencin	It sounds like we are going to take a preliminary view just to see whether we get a consensus with all things included.
Rena Bizios	Should we include the organ as well because it is not one tissue we are talking about but the generation of organs as well.
William Wagner	If you're doing tissue as a sub part of the organ.
David Williams	Cato, can I just make a comment in relation to what Joachim said about restoration, I know there is this term restorative medicine which is being introduced alongside regenerative medicine. Tony Atala is starting with that; he believes that is associated with transplantation, for example face transplantation and I think that is not what we are talking about here. That is the only problem I have with these two. It is likely we get confused with what is the emerging area of restorative medicine. Is that correct Joachim?
Joachim Kohn	That is exactly what I also feared and I fully endorse what you said.
Cato Laurencin	Right, the whole arm transplanters the whole face transplanters, that is a restorative medicine group.
Brendan Harley	Can I offer something to maybe put together because I really like the "renewal and growth," could you think about something like "synthesis, renewal or growth of functional tissue that has been lost due to injury or congenitally."
William Wagner	So "synthesis renewal or growth of functional tissue?"
Joachim Kohn	I think if you just take the word "restoration" out of number two because I think you do not want to have the word restoration in the definition of regeneration, it just isn't right. If you just take two out and say functional renewal or growth by an organism you are in not in bad shape.
Cato Laurencin	Jim?
James Anderson	I was going to follow up on the same statement, take "renewal" out, what does renewal mean?
William Wagner	The term is "regeneration."

James Anderson	It is functional growth of a tissue by an organism. Renewal is either redundant against growth.
Cato Laurencin	I will call the question. This is a pretty good right here for Brendan that seem to have support. What was your beginning?
James Anderson	How do you renew? What is the biologic process of renewal?
Cato Laurencin	I am going to ask if we can call the question because we have our voting things in our hand and this is a current one
William Wagner	This should be where though right?
Cato Laurencin	I think we are there unless we have a burning question.
Hua Ai	I think "synthesis" mostly means chemical; other words should be considered.
Cato Laurencin	The mechanism by which it happens, especially going down to that level of manufacturing or things like that, if that is what you are saying I think that is too detailed for this.
Hua Ai	Yes, you don't see synthesis of organ or tissue.
Cato Laurencin	Yes synthesis is fabricated. Are we ready to vote?
Cato Laurencin	So we're voting for one?
Andrés García	One we're voting for one. I think it's on there, number them.
William Wagner	I think two is redundant...
Cato Laurencin	By show of hands is there interest in adding two to one by anyone, if not we will proceeded with "one" being it.

(d) Final Definition and Voting for "Regeneration"

Regeneration

Synthesis, renewal or growth of new functional tissue which has been lost due to injury, congenital deficiency or has failed due to aging or disease

Voting Yes	47
Voting No	3
Abstain	0
Total Votes	50
Number voting Yes or No	50
Percentage Yes Votes	94%

The definition achieved Consensus, having more than 75% Yes votes, with absolute number greater than 30.

(e) Further Commentary on the Definition of "Regeneration"

In the context that David Williams was given the authority to make minor grammatical alterations, a slightly better wording is as follows; the delegates did not have sufficient time to focus on the grammar in the sentence that was constructed during the course of the discussions in the conference room. It is this which is confirmed to have consensus:

Regeneration

Synthesis, renewal or growth of new functional tissue for use where tissue has failed due to aging or disease, or has been lost through injury, or because of congenital deficiency

B Regenerative Medicine

(a) Possible Definitions of "Regenerative Medicine" Included in Final Program

Therapies that treat disease and injury by the regeneration of functional tissue or organ structures

(b) William Wagner; Perspectives on "Regenerative Medicine" and Suggested Definition

William Wagner	Regenerative medicine, "Therapies that treat disease and injury by the regeneration, which we just defined, of functional tissue or organ structures." Fairly simple straight forward, comments?

Therapies that treat disease and injury by the regeneration of functional tissue or organ structures

(c) Edited Discussion of "Regenerative Medicine"

James Anderson	David, earlier in the previous discussion, you brought up the issue of congenital deformities and I think that should be included but they're not necessarily diseases and not caused by injury. Congenital that's fine…
Nicholas Peppas	Why therapies that treat and not therapy that treats. Why plural, why not singular, therapy the therapy processes?
William Wagner	I guess it is because it's a field. There might be different therapies across the field of regenerative medicine as opposed to one specific approach.
David Williams	Initially I thought you were probably right Nicholas but there will be more than one of them. In my opinion, regenerative medicine includes cell therapy, it includes gene therapy and tissue engineering so there is more than one type, that is why it is plural.
Nicholas Peppas	I agree with you, but it is the definition – "therapy,"
David Williams	You could say just treatment.
Cato Laurencin	I like the fact it is therapy because it is really broad from, for example, ozone therapy, the range is pretty full in terms of the area, there are so many different types of areas.

Brendan Harley	Mine's just a quick point. Compared to what we just added into the previous definition, do we need to also mention aging in this? Because we had mentioned aging specifically in regeneration before.
David Williams	Are you referring to anti-aging therapies?
Brendan Harley	Good idea, I'm just curious whether we should have aging in here because that is another class of loss of function perhaps.
Andrés García	I agree with Brendan if you look at, let's say, osteoarthritis, you can't argue the disease it is just part of getting old. Muscle loss that happens with aging, that's not a disease.
Cato Laurencin	That is not a problem, aging is not a disease.
Andrés García	That's what I am saying, that's exactly what I am saying.
Cato Laurencin	Your bone loss that takes place over time is in a functional range; osteoporosis is not a disease, it is just like you lose some bone.
Andrés García	So there are no conditions that result from aging that are targets for regenerative medicine?
Cato Laurencin	Aging is a natural part of life, the fact is that if you lose bone density, if you lose it to a critical point then that is a disease but if your bone decreases by 1 percent per year, like it does after 40 for all of us, then that is part of life. We are not able to supplement your bone, when you have got a normal range of bone.
David Williams	I think you are absolutely right. I worried about putting "aging" in there. If you look at tissue injury - companies that were involved with skin tissue and injury, most of the time they end up not being able to be cost effective or clinically effective so they go on to cosmetic products. And any company in that area of using skin tissue engineering for cosmetic work they will love that, therefore they can say they are part of medicine. I would like to keep aging out.
Kai Zhang	Why not just remove all the disease stuff so just say therapies that regenerate functional tissue of organ structures.
Cato Laurencin	Good point.
Peter Ma	I was thinking "regenerative medicine" is the therapy itself, what about the science behind it. The science and the therapy.
Cato Laurencin	Unfortunately it has changed over time, yes any other comments? Thoughts? So one suggestion was to say therapies that treat disease by regeneration of functional tissue or organ structures or do the therapies that work by the regeneration of functional tissue or organ structure and leave the other areas out, versus leave them in.
William Wagner	Symmetric with regeneration, that is why we added congenital.
Cato Laurencin	All right is it murmured or keep it in, so we will keep it in. Other comments? Any other comments before we vote? Okay we're ready to vote. it is now open for vote.

(d) Final Definition and Voting for "Regenerative Medicine"

Regenerative Medicine

> **Therapies that treat disease, congenital condition and injury by the regeneration of functional tissue or organ structures**

Voting Yes	44
Voting No	2
Abstain	1
Total Votes	47
Number voting Yes or No	46
Percentage Yes Votes	95.6%

The definition achieved Consensus, having more than 75% Yes votes, with absolute number greater than 30.

(e) Further Commentary on the Definition of "Regenerative Medicine"

In the context that David Williams was given the authority to make minor grammatical alterations, a slightly better wording is as follows; it is this which is confirmed to have consensus:

Regenerative Medicine

> **Therapies that treat disease, congenital conditions or injury by the regeneration of functional tissue or organ structures**

C Tissue Engineering

(a) Possible Definitions of "Tissue Engineering" Included in Final Program

1. The creation of new tissue for the therapeutic reconstruction of the human body, by the deliberate and controlled stimulation of selected target cells through a systematic combination of molecular and mechanical signals[1]
2. The use of a combination of cells, engineering materials, and suitable biochemical factors to improve or replace biological functions in an effort to improve clinical procedures for the repair of damaged tissues and organs[2]

(b) William Wagner; Perspectives on "Tissue Engineering" and Suggested Definition

William Wagner	Okay next we have tissue engineering. Very much talked about, certainly something new since the last consensus conference. A couple of definitions here. One, "the creation of new tissue for the

[1] Williams DF, To engineer is to create; the link between engineering and regeneration, Trends in Biotechnol 2006;24(1):4-8.

[2] www.regenerativemedicine.net.

therapeutic reconstruction of the human body by the deliberate and controlled stimulation of selected target cells through a systematic combination of molecular or mechanical signals." That is from David Williams' paper in Trends in Biotechnology article you referenced earlier, and then from regenerativemedicine.net "the use of a combination of cells, engineering materials and suitable biochemical factors to improve or replace biological functions in an effort to improve clinical outcomes for the repair of damaged tissues and organs" Those of us in the field certainly have probably seen a million times that graphic with the cells, the materials and the biochemical factors and then that label tissue engineering so I think that is consistent at least with number two and with number one as well, although number two is a little bit more synced on that.

(c) Edited Discussion of "Tissue Engineering"

Peter Ma	My comment on this is that it is not necessary to use all of these - because we may use cells, tissues, signals all together, but maybe some of them. So the tissue engineers may use one or multiple things, but it is not necessary to have to have all three components.
Elizabeth Cosgriff-H	Even if it is endogenous or exogenous cells, it still has cells as part of it, so it doesn't necessarily preclude the combination in this. I think the traditional tissue engineering paradigm is all three. You don't have to add all three in the construct.
Arthur Coury	Thank you, I go counter to almost all my colleagues. I think in my statement and my belief of what tissue engineering is. Here is my definition, "Exerting systematic control of the body's cells, matrices, and or fluids for desired therapeutic outcomes."
Arthur Coury	What is a tissue expander? Does it use cells? Well, probably engineering material, probably, but does it use biochemical factors? Does it do that? What is an anti-adhesion device that regenerates, that allows healing to occur? Most people would say that is not tissue engineering, but I say that it is, because you will see a completely normal surface after all of this.
Arthur Coury	I keep engineering in there, but I don't specify why.
Peter Ma	Let me get back on that question again. For example, you may do tissue engineering by delivering signals, you may never deliver a signal there. They are repaired, is this tissue engineering or not? Could be just the way a factor works. Could be the body, you already have the cells and everything else. Just as one signal is weak, you add that signal. You didn't add additional cells or increase additional cells, then it worked. Or you have other needed things already in the body.

Peter Ma	The only thing we need is a structural component. You need a scaffold to give shape. You put that in there. Now it's regenerating the tissue with that structure. So I think there is a possibility for us to use one or multiple components, but not necessarily everything else has to be used.
Rena Bizios	I don't feel any disagreement with you, Peter and with Elizabeth. Still the triad of tissue engineering are the cells, are the materials, are the stimuli or factors, if we want to call them factors. I prefer the stimuli because biochemicals can be factors, but we need to bring in the biophysical stimuli as well.
Rena Bizios	And what Art said a little bit earlier, for me, is a little bit more appropriate for the last part of this definition, which here states, "To improve clinical procedures, etc." Perhaps that can be rephrased to include some of the suggestions of Art, but I don't hear any different between you and what Elizabeth said.
Timmie Topoleski	Cato, this is the first time I've seen the phrase "In an effort to," in the definition because it sounds like, "We're going to try, but we don't know." I would recommend that we get rid of that phrase just to say what we're really doing here.
Cato Laurencin	Okay. That's a good comment. Other comments?
Xingdong Zhang	We have to answer whether tissue engineering is a technology or discipline . . . So this part, okay, we have asked what is tissue engineering? It is technology or discipline?
Cato Laurencin	It is a discipline focused on the combination of cells, engineering, which are immutable facts. Is that what you're saying?
Xingdong Zhang	Okay.
David Williams	Okay, I am not necessarily defending number one, but there is a point about number two, and I agree with you about "In an effort" I perfectly understand that. But "To improve clinical procedures," rather implies for me the syntax that you are taking one clinical procedure and you are going to improve that. Much of tissue engineering is in fact a very different clinical approach. I am just worried about the English, the syntax to "improve clinical procedures" means that you are going to improve an existing procedure by doing that.
Deon Bezuidenhout	I was just wondering if the problem of using all three or just combinations of one or two of the triangles vertices can be obviated by using "suitable combinations" of the three and that could be the one or two or three.
Cato Laurencin	Suitable combinations.
David Williams	I agree with that.
Elizabeth Cosgriff-H	I just want to reiterate Rena's statement of making the biochemical factors to be broader to biological cues or stimuli. I think is what

	she also said. I think that's important that we get away from just biochemical.
Rena Bizios	I like the biochemical and the biophysical because there are two different entities and people have to be aware we have two different categories. I won't mind one extra word there, however. I would go back to the engineering materials. My suggestion is they will be either engineered materials, or because we have naturally occurring materials, which are used for tissue engineering applications, we have to say natural or synthetic materials. Or something appropriate to cover both categories of materials which are used for tissue engineering.
Bikramjit Basu	I would like to replace this "engineering materials" by "scaffolds." Because most of this tissue engineering is essentially based on the scaffolds. So if we can mention in engineering materials as far as scaffolds, that would be . . . a nice addition.
Carl Simon	Going along with what Art was saying, to make it more generalized, you could say something like, "To effect desirable clinical outcomes." That way you don't have to say exactly what it is you're trying to do, but we all know we want to do good.
Brendan Harley	I wanted to emphasize what Carl was saying, because there are many new flavors of tissue engineering that we have seen over recent years. Cancer tissue engineering, for example. We are not trying to grow a cancer to put in a patient, but we are applying the principles of tissue engineering to study a process, sometimes even outside the body, and that never goes into the body. That would also apply to drug testing. Systems I think we can be forward thinking. I think it is getting back to what Professor Zhang is asking. Is this a paradigm, or a process as opposed to an outcome? I think that would be really important to clarify at the end.
Laura Poole-Warren	I was going to suggest that rather than use "engineering materials" we actually use "biomaterials."
Cato Laurencin	All right. Other comments?
Rena Bizios	It said "Functions to improve clinical outcomes" instead of going "Functions in an effort to improve" . . .
Cato Laurencin	I think everyone is okay with that, we are moving in an effort. All right, so we have two. We are taking one of them?
William Wagner	I tried to put into number two. The key things, is there anything you think I am missing from one or the discussion that is not here? Again trying to keep it general.
Cato Laurencin	Yes.
Yunbing Wang	I agree with Peter Ma's opinion, because for tissue engineering, traditional people think this is a three combination: cells, biomaterials, and factors. But, today it does not mean we have to

	do that. For some new technology we just use materials to induce by the control the structures. That should also be done through part of tissue engineering. So for this one, I also think the combination … we must have another selection.
Cato Laurencin	I had a definition before. The definition I have used before says "alone or in combination," just to make it very clear. These are used in tissue engineering paradigms, "the use alone or in combination of cells, materials, and biological factors."
Peter Ma	That is how it is with me. Alone or in combination as the same means either of them or a combination of them. I also want to comment about cancer tissue engineering. I think here generally we think that tissue engineering is a therapy to treat disease or lost tissues. I think those constructs could be used as a model for our disease studies, but not what we think as tissue engineering itself. Maybe they call this tissue engineering, the way to make a cancer model. I don't consider that tissue engineering.
Jiandong Ding	I think that the term tissue or organ should appear in that definition, otherwise it is not really tissue engineering. Because we have deleted this very important key word.
William Wagner	Yes that's a good point because the biomaterial if it is alone it is just a medical device that would be like a stent which would not be tissue engineering.
Cato Laurencin	Improve or replace biological tissues? Or biological functions? Instead of biological function, biological tissue?
Yunbing Wang	Maybe we could use some combination, all combination of cells, biomaterials, and chemical effectors. In that case we can use two or use three of them.
Cato Laurencin	It says alone or in combination. I think that hits it. Other questions, comments?
Hanry Yu	Besides mechanical factors or stimuli, in fact there are other types, electrical and such. So, it's better to use physical or biophysical factors rather than mechanical only.
Cato Laurencin	Tissue engineering, by definition does not have that. So you are adding that in.
Hanry Yu	It is replacing the mechanical with physical or biophysical.
Cato Laurencin	Okay. Are we ready to take a stab at voting? Are we ready?
William Wagner	Just voting on two?
Cato Laurencin	Yes, voting on two.
Elizabeth Cosgriff-H	I think the first "improve" is redundant. So "in combination to replace" and take out "that improve." Or just "generate new tissue?"
William Wagner	Sometimes you're augmenting.

David Williams	I think in number two as it stands now, I see there is a problem there because that could, if it is biomaterials alone, be an implantable medical device such as a hip replacement.
Peter Ma	But that is not creating tissues. If you put "creating tissue" in there that concern is gone, right?
David Williams	Well it could be a porous coated hip replacement, where you are creating tissue at the interface to stabilize it.
Cato Laurencin	Some people actually call that tissue engineering, though.
David Williams	Wrongly.
Cato Laurencin	At any case, other comments.
Cato Laurencin	Let us take a stab at voting on it. Are we going to vote on number two alone? Are we ready to vote? Yes?

(d) Final Definition and Voting for "Tissue Engineering"

Tissue Engineering

The use of cells, biomaterials and suitable molecular or physical factors, alone or in combination, to repair or replace tissue to improve clinical outcomes

Voting Yes	40
Voting No	5
Abstain	1
Total Votes	46
Number voting Yes or No	45
Percentage Yes Votes	88.8%

The definition achieved Consensus, having more than 75% Yes votes, with absolute number greater than 30.

D Regenerative Engineering

(a) Possible Definitions of "Regenerative Engineering" Included in Final Program

None was included as the term was not on the original list of terms to be discussed.

(b) Cato Laurencin; Perspectives on "Regenerative Engineering" and Suggested Definition

| Cato Laurencin | We have had tissue engineering now over a quarter of a century and there has always been a discussion over how we can do more to progress the field. We have had some wins here in terms of tissue engineering, but also some disappointments in terms of wide spread use in terms of technology that we have had. In a couple of meetings, we have started to talk about the possibilities in areas beyond many of the traditional areas of tissue engineering. With |

Jim Anderson and Art Coury and others, we got together in 2010 where we said what are the grand challenges and what are the new ways that we can think about fields and what are the fields that can prompt grand challenges.

Cato Laurencin   The concept is how can we bring other fields that may be relevant to move to the next level of this area and really converge those fields together. At the same time the concept of convergence came to the floor. This is put forth by Phil Sharp, talking about how the life science, the physical science of engineering brought together for pursuing different areas, could be important.

Cato Laurencin   There's a convergence book that came out. At the National Academy of Science, Nick Peppas and I were on the committee to put together the book. Convergence means the coming together of insights and approaches from originally distinct fields and bringing them together.

Cato Laurencin   We looked at the elephant in the room in tissue regeneration and the fact that new strategies and a new ecosystem were needed for moving to the next generation. That new ecosystem includes scientists, engineers, clinicians, lay people bringing a new ecosystem together.

Cato Laurencin   We have talked about science and transitional medicine. We have talked about the future of tissue regeneration, which we felt lies in regenerative engineering with biomaterials playing an important role. The definition that we have had is the convergence of what is new over the last fifteen to twenty years that can be brought together to bear to be able to work together for regeneration. Advanced material science in terms of biomaterials. Stem cell science. Physics and physical forces. Developmental biology, which we believe is very important in clinical translation. Patient factors. Clinical factors in determining regeneration of complex tissues, organs, and organ systems.

Cato Laurencin   We have thought about this and if you could think about designing something like this and moving forward a field, the first thing we decided is we needed to define the field in a way that comes to a firm definition, define some of the strategies behind this area, and also define the ecosystem that surrounds the area in building the new field. We were thinking about this from the ground up.

Cato Laurencin   Areas of advanced materials, stem cell science, physics, physical forces, bioreactors, developmental biology, how a salamander regenerates, and also clinical factors and getting clinicians involved is a part of it because one person may have a problem, may have four or five different types of solutions depending on the person. Depending on their immunology. Depending on the patient factors. It leads to this definition that's there.

Cato Laurencin   One of the areas that we are talking about is developmental biology. We can create limbs in salamanders without doing any of the amputations, by just implanting factors that take place during regeneration. Purifying and placing them we can actually create limbs from scratch in animals. It is easy to do it when you cut off an arm, but creating a brand-new limb from scratch using the factors that come from different mammals. These sorts of technologies, we think, are going to be important in this next generation in terms of bringing developmental biology into the regeneration theme.

Cato Laurencin   Since our paper in Science Translational Medicine, we have got a book on Regenerative Engineering that is out. Then we have a new journal of regenerative engineering that tries to bring these areas together.

Cato Laurencin   We just started a new society called the Regenerative Engineering Society. Again, clinicians, scientists, engineers, lay people brought together to be able to work on it. Also, it is good in this ecosystem to create a common definition. One of the things that we have got is a number of definitions for regenerative medicine because we have people who are working, clinicians that think that they are board certified in regenerative medicine.

Cato Laurencin   I was in Beijing last week with President Xi Jinping who addressed us at the Great Hall. He said we have to take leap frog views. We have to think about in the future. We have to take leap frog views and think about how we can create technologies and sciences and ways of thinking that can actually ... not just move us incrementally but can give us a leap frog view in terms of how we can move forward. We believe that in terms of regeneration, this may be able to do it.

Cato Laurencin   The clinical end is very important. How we can create an ecosystem with clinicians is an example that actually talks about the fact that you have to have clinicians as part of it because there are patient factors that are involved.

Cato Laurencin   Then finally, this new strategy in ecosystem is needed. Looking at convergence of engineering, life sciences, translational medicine, bringing them together in terms of patient care. With common terminology, common strategies, we think the field can move forward fairly fast in terms of people that are like minded being able to create these areas of regenerative engineering.

Cato Laurencin   Finally, this is a proposed workshop that's going to be taking place in October by the National Academy of Medicine and National Academy of Sciences on regenerative engineering and looking at how regenerative engineering in terms of bringing in areas such as developmental biology, immunology, stem cell science, and how it

| | also focuses on patient factors in making decisions regarding treatment can become very useful in deciding what happens with patient variability and of outcomes when regenerative treatments are performed. |
| Cato Laurencin | This is the definition: "Convergence of advanced material science, stem cell science, physics, developmental biology, and clinical translation toward the re generational complex tissues, organs, and organ systems." |

(c) Edited Discussion of "Regenerative Engineering"

Editor's note: A wide-ranging discussion took place in Session III around the broad but new subject of regenerative engineering. In Session III, the resulting vote was inconclusive; a further discussion took place during the Final General Summary Session, and a further vote was taken. These two discussions are included here in Part One and Part Two, respectively.

PART ONE: Discussion in Session III

Rena Bizios	I like this pretty good definition very much. The only question I have, why isn't chemistry involved in there? There is a lot of chemistry going on in all of this aspect. In your definition you put physics. I agree. The materials, the stem cells, exclusively a very good choice, and developmental biology. Any particular reason that chemistry is not included? Is it implied in the other ones? Isn't it important in this context?
Cato Laurencin	I think there is some implication of this in advanced material science.
Rena Bizios	Not only in that. It is in the stem cells in terms of production of chemical compounds, the effect of chemical compounds on them, the developmental biology has a lot of chemical aspects involved.
Joachim Kohn	I would like to express my excitement about what you are doing. It' is very innovative and it is not only useful, it is very much needed. The definition that you have is also, I think, very well rounded. I think that the idea of including chemistry explicitly may be something you want to consider. Generally, I think this is really exciting stuff. Thank you for bringing it forward.
Hua Ai	I think it is tough to define which one is complex and which is not complex and to draw the line. Which tissue is a complex tissue? Maybe it is possible to remove "complex?"
Bikramjit Basu	I would like to propose the "convergence of biomaterial science" instead of "advanced material science." And, to combine physics and chemistry together, perhaps we can use the word "natural sciences."
Cato Laurencin	The point about the material sciences is that when we look at where we are, we have a lot of great things taking place in material

	science, that we did not have fifteen to twenty years ago. Part of that is this concept, and it speaks to what Rena is saying, is that it speaks to the fact that we now understand how the chemistry of the material can dictate the cell behavior that is taking place.
Cato Laurencin	The other concern is that when you have a number of different areas and you become so diffused then someone says what are you really? What are your emphasis areas? As a field, we do not take any area and say you can't be a part of it. The emphasis is convergence, what are the two biggest emphasis areas?
David Williams	Cato, let me first say that I recognize the work you are doing, you and your group. I think it is as Joachim said, a very good projection for the future. I think it is very important.
David Williams	I would have to put on record a slight concern about the definition itself. As I said this morning, I do not like definitions which start off with "the field of" and I really do not like like "the convergence of." To go along with what Rena said, you have advanced material sciences, stem cell sciences, physics, developmental biology, and then the clinical translation. Yes, there's no chemistry. There's no word "engineering" in there. Once you go down the route of giving some examples then you run the real risk of leaving things out which are equally important. I am just putting it on the record. I have to say that.
David Williams	As I said this morning about Bob Langer's definition of tissue engineering, that was a good start. What I would suggest to you is to use this as a start. That will evolve over a few years to have, perhaps, more of a constructive and specific definition for it.
William Wagner	Question. Could you contrast regenerative medicine and regenerative engineering? Is it that regenerative engineering is defined here as a discipline? And we have defined regenerative medicine as a therapeutic approach? Or, am I interpreting that wrong?
Cato Laurencin	I think a couple things. One is that the concept of convergence, that the belief is that it is really bringing together these different technologies that are going to be making a difference rather than, say, ozone therapy is the cure all. In regenerative medicine, someone could say I place them in an ozone chamber for a half hour and I cure your problems. That is number one.
Cato Laurencin	The second is that this has identified a certain set of areas that we believe will be important for being able to achieve leap frog types of view.
Cato Laurencin	The third is that the concept of clinical translation, and we understood now that there is a fairly big emphasis on this. If you look at the variability of outcomes, of different types of engineered materials, the clinical factor and immunology of the patient

	actually makes a very big difference. The clinical translation part of the downstream part becomes very important part of the process.
Kai Zhang	Yes, Cato. I agree with both what David and Bill just said. People will ask this question once we start defining what regenerative engineering is. What is the difference among tissue engineering, regenerative medicine and regenerative engineering. We need to definitely make it clear the regenerative engineering is different from the other two perspectives. By reading what we have defined here, I couldn't tell clearly.
Cato Laurencin	I think that the elements are, number one, the concept of the convergence approach which is something new over the last ten years. The fact of bringing together insights and bringing together technologies that are disparate. We do not talk about "alone" or "in combination." We talk about really bringing together, technologies that are disparate that are really brought to be able to treat the area.
Cato Laurencin	The second is the area of developmental biology and clinical translation which I think are areas that are not talked about that much in terms of how we traditionally think about those areas of tissue engineering.
Rena Bizios	I agree with Cato's comments. For me, the big difference is the stem cells exclusively used. In regenerative medicine so far, and I believe in the future, because of this combination with the clinical translation, the stem cells are going to be the ones that are going to be used almost exclusively. We are using cells from all kinds of other sources, we are using stem cells, too, but here it is exclusive.
Rena Bizios	Last, I like the word "advanced materials" because we have to stop thinking of different materials. Perhaps on different aspects of those materials which have been used for all kinds of applications, implant applications. Including the clinical tissue engineering applications. For me, those are the key words in addition to what Cato said regarding that emphasis on clinical translation.
Jian Ji	I personally like this definition very much. I think it is good to combine advanced materials, stem cells, and the other things together. I think the final goal for the regenerative engineering is for the application. Could we add also fabrication. Fabrication technology, because when we need to put the materials, stem cells, and the biology things together, the new fabrication technology is really important to put them together.
Cato Laurencin	I think it is a very important point. We are now partnering with the Advanced Regenerative Manufacturing Institute, the new institute that was created by President Obama, and we have become their key organizational partner moving forward because of the fact that, in this area of regeneration, we believe that

	biomanufacturing is really important, even scale up in biomanufacturing is important.
Arthur Coury	If there is an improved definition, I can't see how we could get around the consideration of pharmacology as being really important. It is about three times or four times the size of the medical-device industry, and I think leaving it out could be offensive to some of our colleagues that are in that field.
William Wagner	I want to move forward with a vote here. You're the champion of this. Did you hear anything that you feel needs change?
Cato Laurencin	I think that I could take it two ways. One is I think that the pharmacology consideration is something that we should think about. I am not sure we should put it in this definition, but I think that it's worthy during the next year. To discuss it, and think about which way do we go with it. On the biomanufacturing, again, I do believe it's important.
Cato Laurencin	I think that will be something, too, that we would think about for incorporating over the next year to two years, but in terms of where we are now, I think that this is where we would like to foresee consensus.
William Wagner	Okay, so with no edits, I am calling the vote for this term as defined. Are we ready for the votes?
Cato Laurencin	Yes.
William Wagner	Yes, ready to vote.

(d) Final Definition and Voting for "Regenerative Engineering"

Regenerative Engineering

The convergence of advanced materials sciences, stem cell sciences, physics, developmental biology and clinical translation for the regeneration of complex tissue and organ systems

Voting Yes	19
Voting No	25
Abstain	2
Total Votes	46
Number voting Yes or No	44
Percentage Yes Votes	43.2%

The definition achieved neither consensus nor provisional consensus.

PART TWO: Discussion in Final Session

David Williams	I am just going to introduce this and ask Cato to make some more comments. We had an extensive discussion yesterday and Cato presented some slides. This is a relatively new, not absolutely new,

but a relatively new concept. And one of the objectives of this consensus conference was to look at new concepts and new terms. We did not achieve consensus. In fact we didn't get to provisional consensus yesterday. But it is such an important area. I spoke to Cato last night, and said there were several reasons why I think it did not get to that vote.

David Williams   I think one of them was a confusion about the difference between this and regenerative medicine, maybe even tissue engineering. I am not sure that we all understood that one. So I thought it would be sensible for us to discuss that. But I did say to Cato, he could not come back with exactly the same definition, for us to consider and vote on. So I asked him to make a change or changes.

David Williams   So Cato gave me this a short while ago, with a change adding "engineering" to the definition. And he put that there as engineered regeneration. In other words, the engineering is not within the various sciences which are converging, but it is lower down in engineered regeneration.

David Williams   So I would like a further discussion. Cato, I am going to ask for a general discussion, do you want to add to that at the moment?

Cato Laurencin   Yes, so I think there, was whether we could make changes. And I thought that there was a pretty good consensus before we voted, so I said okay no, let us just keep it as it is and move forward. But it didn't have consensus. So I am absolutely happy to see if there are changes that people think that need to be made, to introduce the changes there. And one that was there, was talking about the fact that one of the distinctions should be adding engineering to it. So, "engineered regeneration of complex tissue and organ systems" is added.

Cato Laurencin   The other was, I guess there was a question about regenerative medicine versus regenerative engineering. I thought about this. This was a consensus adopted definition of regenerative medicine, "therapy to treat disease, congenital condition and injury, by regeneration of functional tissue organ systems." It's sort of an all-inclusive catch all in terms of this area of regeneration. But regenerative engineering differs in the emphasis on engineering principles, and this emphasis of convergence which is a new approach where we bring together new technologies and new ways of thinking.

David Williams   Thank you Cato. We will have broad discussion about that.

Peter Ma   I think it is really an important area, so we should have this in some way defined. I really think that this, in a way is different from the regenerative medicine. This is emphasizing engineering. The other side, the regenerative medicine comes from the stem cell terms, more from the biological aspect although they use the materials as a support. In regenerative engineering, the material is more designed, to engineer the stem cell environment, to allow the stem cells to function. So that is what, from my understanding, this might be more from the engineering aspect, how to create that environment, make tissue engineering happen.

David Williams   Thank you. Mario? Mario has an, I think, interesting point here.

Mário Barbosa   I don't know if I am going to mention the interesting point you are actually referring to. But anyway, I'm referring to the word of "convergence." For me, "integration" is stronger, in the sense that different disciplines actually integrate to produce new technologies. The interesting aspect that David was referring about, that I will also mention, is that in my university where we have a bioengineering master's degree for over ten years, and the students compete with students from medicine with very high entry marks. We had to replace regenerative medicine, by regenerative engineering, because the doctors were opposed to the first phrase. It actually corresponds more to what we are doing, it is engineering, rather than medicine. The other thing that I would like to mention is about the need to include all those sciences. For me, materials science and biology would be the key ingredients. I don't know if you need to put physics, chemistry and other aspects, because I think this dilutes the importance of material science and biology.

David Williams   Thank you Mario. I have to say I like the integration concept, I mentioned to Cato, and I mentioned it here yesterday, a definition starting off with "convergent," I don't like that myself. "Integration," I believe is far better. That is just my view.

Rena Bizios   The enumeration of all these fields is very good, we can add one and subtract another one, fine with me. However, the addition of all these things, they are not equal to engineering, because the principles of engineering are very important, and here is an example, bioreactors. All kinds of other aspects of characterizing, they are advanced materials, yes exactly. The word engineering here is for me, and I think I'm going to put it after advanced materials science and engineering and then stem cells, we have to get the engineering word there. Thank you.

Frank Witte   Yes, I think it is an important term, that we at least have to address and somehow define today. I am just looking at our center for regenerative therapies in Berlin, and we have about a hundred PhD students, and so for the last two years I saw with all the proposals and presentations, more and more the word regenerative engineering. And in this interdisciplinary field, at least we have to think about how to define what it basically means, because it will be used among these young researchers more and more in the future.

David Williams   Thank you, Frank. Anybody else? Kai?

Kai Zhang	I too also think, the engineering is very important. And I agree with Peter and several others, this is an important concept, because there are many engineers actually in this room. So I would add the engineering, one word, engineering principles. To the definition, I don't know, because it is not only engineering, there are maybe others.
David Williams	I don't think it is only engineering principles, it is engineering practices as well. And I do not think we will go too long. I think the word "engineering" is sufficiently instructive for us to use it like that.
Laura Poole-Warren	I have a suggestion, because I think that including various disciplines in there you are always in danger of including too many or excluding some, and I am wondering whether we could go along the lines of a "multidisciplinary approach to engineering technologies for regeneration of complex tissues and organs."
David Williams	I personally think that's taken away the edge of putting some of these different disciplines in.
Laura Poole-Warren	Because I think you could have a footnote in terms of "this may include a range of different disciplines." But I think the fact is, is that if you don't list all the disciplines, you're going to be missing out on some.
David Williams	Cato, that would be a fundamental change of definitions if we did that.
Cato Laurencin	Certainly to a great extent it is. One of the thought processes involved in this is looking at where we were twenty years from now, twenty years ago to now. And what are some of the areas we have in our inventory now that we have not had before? In terms of advanced materials and nanotechnology? The power of stem cells, into only being able to differentiate, but the immunological effects. And then also integrating developmental biology which we have not done before. And finally, the patient factors involving clinical translation and determining outcomes.
Peter Ma	That is where the definition is going, the term is too broad. Because we are talking about medicine. In some other fields, like water resources, they are also talking about the regeneration of the water resources. So whether we should add, define biomedical engineering or medical engineering.
David Williams	I personally don't think so. Does anybody agree with that, I think we are probably in a good shape there.
Arthur Coury	I mentioned yesterday that I think leaving pharmacology out of there is leaving a big factor out of there. And if we are modifying it, at this point I think I would recommend adding that.
David Williams	Okay, Art is suggesting including pharmacology. I think we are getting concerned about having too many disciplines in there. Do

	you think the pharmacology aspect is almost included in clinical translation?
James Anderson	My comment was, do we really need the term "complex" in front of tissues. I mean the organ is a fairly complex tissue, at least I thought it was.
Cato Laurencin	I definitely yield to Jim on that, I think that originally when this had been developed and discussed, the ability to be able to address grand challenges and to address things at a complex, or bringing together these technologies is what was the thought.
David Williams	I can understand that, and sometimes addressing a grand challenge, or NIH, you have to put in some rather emotive terms. But that doesn't mean to say we have to have them in our definitions. That is in your footnote to your agencies.
Cato Laurencin	Agreed.
Serena Best	I just wonder whether the clinical translation is the aim, rather than one in the list of disciplines.
David Williams	Do you mean after developmental biology you could put in, for the clinical translation?
Serena Best	I would have thought that's the aim.
Cato Laurencin	Yes, one of the concepts is that in all of these disciplines, the clinician and patient factors are so important. And so whether you created a ... so integrating patient factors that are involved in terms of making the clinical decision, even using a treatment, is something that is becoming more and more important. We talk about ecosystem, we would like to have something that not only involves engineers and scientists, but also clinicians. And so that is why the feeling has been, and the discussion has been, that this is an integral part. As one of the components of it, not just the endpoint.
John Brash	I'm wondering if we need that "advanced" in front of "materials?"
David Williams	I think this is because we are forward looking. I think in the materials science area, generally, and not just chemistry, but in the materials science area, there is such a thing as advanced materials science. And I think probably, looking at this forward-looking concept, it is better to include it there. That's my view. Anybody that would like to take it out? Kam? One says take it out, two says take it out, three, four. If your hands aren't up, I am saying leave it in. We leave it in, sorry.
Nicholas Peppas	The term has been word-smithed a lot. It's very well done, it's balanced, it includes the main terms that we use at the National Academy when we described convergence. You cannot do regenerative engineering without all these terms. I heard what you said Art, I would tend to say pharmacology isn't included. I mean it is important, but it doesn't have the same impact as the other terms. I would be very happy if we proceed with this term as it is.

David Williams	Thank you Nick, I will take maybe two or three more comments. It has been important to have this extensive discussion. Which will be in the text to support Cato's vision, if we get provisional consensus. Do I see any hands up here, to carry on forward? No. It was still on this definition, before we take a vote, any further comments, maybe suggestions of change.
John Brash	I'm wondering about "physics," might not that be covered already by "engineering," I don't think we mean by "physics" quantum physics or nuclear physics or anything like that, the physics presumably meant to be included here is kind of like classical physics, which would be covered by engineering I believe.
David Williams	I was thinking more of biophysics.
John Brash	That's classical physics.
David Williams	Okay, we'll take John's comment, do we need physics in there? Do we need physics if we have engineering? Comments on that. Joachim?
Joachim Kohn	Yes, I would like to comment that we need the physics in there, it is distinct from engineering in my opinion, I think I like it very much like it is.
David Williams	You have lost, Jim?
James Anderson	Yes, I always thought that engineering was applied physics, I think it can be removed.
David Williams	That's two. Any stronger view on this. Mario?
Mário Barbosa	Going to my previous point, I mean if we put too many items there, we remove strength of some of them. I do not think that we need physics. So in order to increase the strength of the other aspects, I would remove physics, because in part, it is already included in engineering. In my view.
David Williams	Okay that is a reasonably strong view, but I am going to take a show of hands here, before we get to a definition. So first of all, and the choice will be, as you have it now, with physics and engineering, or without physics. I think we all agree engineering has to be there. So those who would like to keep it as is now with both physics and engineering, show your hand. Those who would like to delete physics. That has it, so we will delete physics. Okay, I think we have a good definition. I think we can take a vote on that. Wait a second before we get it right. Ready to go.

(e) Final Definition and Voting for "Regenerative Engineering"

Regenerative Engineering

The integration of advanced materials sciences, stem cell science, engineering, developmental biology and clinical translation for the regeneration of complex tissue and organ systems

Voting Yes	31
Voting No	18
Abstain	1
Total Votes	50
Number voting Yes or No	49
Percentage Yes Votes	63.3%

The version of the definition achieved Provisional Consensus, having more than 50% Yes votes.

E Decellularization

(a) Possible Definitions of "Decellularization" Included in Final Program

The processing of tissues or organs that removes cells, leaving the functional and structural proteins of the extracellular matrix as a scaffold

(b) William Wagner; Perspectives on "Decellularization" and Suggested Definition

William Wagner	Decellularization. We have a definition here. "The processing of tissues, or organs, to remove cells and cellular debris, with the aim of preserving biological activity and structural integrity of the extracellular matrix as a scaffold."

(c) Edited Discussion of "Decellularization"

Rena Bizios	Should we mention something that these are the native cells or something like that to specify that the cells already exist in those tissues, and they are part of the extracellular matrix. Or is it clear by just the statement as it appears now?
William Wagner	I think it would be very unlikely that you would think that you would get a tissue, or organ, and put cells in and then … I think the simplicity, to me, it's pretty obvious what cell is there.
John Ramshaw	The question I have is in structural integrity because I know one laboratory I read they make a paste out of their decellularized tissue and use that for injections and so forth. That's decellularized, but not retaining structural integrity.
William Wagner	You said they make a paste from their decellularized tissue.
John Ramshaw	Yes.
William Wagner	You are right. They do. They process it into hydrogel; they do other things, but the decellularization process is something that is being studied and utilized now quite a bit in the biomaterials community.

Cato Laurencin	I guess the only question, would it be "and/or structural integrity?" There may be some that you just want the old lattice. You will take all the materials out just to have a lattice work. Some of the people were doing the whole arm, or are doing a face transplant where they take all the cells out, take all the materials out, all it has, it doesn't have any activity at all. They don't want to have any activity, they just want to have the structural integrity that looks like a face. Yes?
Deon Bezuidenhout	Just to answer Rena's point. There are actually people who engineer tissues in vitro and then decellularize them and use the scaffolds again. Simon Hoerstrup does that in Zurich. Then, a second a point. I do not believe that decellularization is always done to preserve the biological activity because they are also used, for instance, in bioprosthetic heart valves, where the goal is not to tissue engineer, but just to have a function of tissue. I am not sure if the definition is 100% correct.
Kam Leong	Have you considered confluent cell layer? A tissue or something? I thought one of the most useful methodologies, just the growth of cells on tissue culture polystyrene or something, get to a confluent layer and get rid of the cells, then I do have a useful decellularized matrix.
William Wagner	Right, so that would be a tissue, right?
William Wagner	I am thinking of Laura Niklason, this is probably the best example with the generated blood vessel and then decellularization; I would consider that is a tissue that she generates.
William Wagner	Generally when the term decellularization is being used, as I have seen in the literature many times, it is with this eye towards preserving the biological activity and avoiding harsh crosslinking protocols.
William Wagner	The decellularized tissues, or the ECM-based materials, as opposed to the glutaraldehyde fixed, or older technologies, I could say, is that you want to preserve the bioactivity. You want to preserve the cell recognition, and the growth factor, some amount of growth factor there and reduce immunogenicity at the same time. But you sacrifice the long term structural integrity to do that. You recognize that it is going to remodel now when you put it in, in vivo.
David Williams	Bill, I understand exactly what you're saying there, but I do not think we can disregard what Deon said because decellularization of bovine pericardium, for example, is still a hugely important component of bioprosthetic valves and other devices. I think here we have to have "and/or." We have to allow for both under decellularization, because in those situations, it is not being used as a scaffold.
Cato Laurencin	Yes, we have the example of the Restore device, whether you like it or not, the intestinal submucosa device that is used for the

	shoulder. It is decellularized. Everything's taken out, and you try to make it as inert as possible and nonbiologically active as possible. It is only used for structural integrity.
Peter Ma	I am also wondering about preserving biological activities. I think that is hard to do, actually. You can maybe preserve in some way.
William Wagner	Yes, I didn't intend for it to mean entire, just implies preserved some biological activity.
Cato Laurencin	I think when he is saying, preserved biological activity, it means preserved to some extent. From zero to zero plus, or whatever.
Peter Ma	Okay.
Cato Laurencin	Okay. Other questions? David?
David Williams	You could just remove "as a scaffold," at the end. That would encompass both types.
Cato Laurencin	Right. Good point.
Cato Laurencin	Everybody ready to vote? Okay. Open to vote.

(d) Final Definition and Voting for "Decellularization"

Decellularization

The processing of tissues or organs to remove cells and cellular debris, with the aim of preserving biological activity and/or structural integrity of the extracellular matrix

Voting Yes	44
Voting No	5
Abstain	0
Total Votes	49
Number voting Yes or No	49
Percentage Yes Votes	89.8%

The definition achieved Consensus, having more than 75% Yes votes, with absolute number greater than 30.

F Recellularization

(a) Possible Definitions of "Recellularization" Included in Final Program

The repopulation of decellularized tissues or organs by functional cells

(b) William Wagner; Perspectives on "Recellularization" and Suggested Definition

William Wagner	Certainly in the literature is this notion of decellularizing tissues, preserving bioactivity, not fixing, or minimally fixing, and then re-populating, often with iPS cells, although that is not part of the

requirement. The re-popularization of decellularized tissues, or organs, by cells with the objective of ultimately re-introducing functional activity, whatever that may be. My suggestion is:

Recellularization
The repopulation of decellularized tissues or organs by cells with the objective of ultimately reintroducing functional activity

(c) Edited Discussion of "Recellularization"

There was no discussion of this definition

(d) Final Definition and Voting for "Recellularization"

Recellularization

The repopulation of decellularized tissues or organs by cells with the objective of ultimately reintroducing functional activity

Voting Yes	42
Voting No	2
Abstain	1
Total Votes	45
Number voting Yes or No	44
Percentage Yes Votes	95.4%

The definition achieved Consensus, having more than 75% Yes votes, with absolute number greater than 30.

G Whole Organ Engineering

(a) Possible Definitions of "Whole Organ Engineering" Included in Final Program

The engineering of replacement organs by the decellularization and subsequent recellularization of donor organs, that results in the preservation of tissue type specific matrix in a 3D architecture that closely mimics the native tissue and maintains the natural vasculature network

(b) William Wagner; Perspectives on "Whole Organ Engineering" and Suggested Definition

Whole Organ Engineering
The engineering of replacement organs by the decellularization and subsequent recellularization of donor organs, that results in the preservation of tissue type specific matrix in a 3D architecture that closely mimics the native tissue, and with recellularization seeks to provide organ-specific functionality

(c) Edited Discussion of "Whole Organ Engineering"

Rena Bizios	The obtaining of replacement organs is important, we have to write something it. "Obtain," or some other verb statement there before the replacement. It's not only the engineering, but you have to obtain it, to get it, to formulate it.
William Wagner	Okay. The donor organs are what you are operating on, right? The donor organs is how you are getting the replacement organ.
Andrés García	Is decellularization the only way to make a whole organ? Getting rid of the cells and then adding the new cells? Why couldn't somebody come up with a fancy bioprinter and print a kidney?
William Wagner	Yes, that's absolutely correct. It is the same. I think it falls into the same category as biomaterial. Is a biological material not a biomaterial? To a lot of people outside of this room, that is a biomaterial. Our position is, "No, we are going to make this definition that defines a biomaterial as a specific subset."
William Wagner	Whole-organ engineering is a term that is being used routinely now by those in the field that are doing this decellularization-recellularization. The whole-organ aspect is a little bit different. Other people are saying, 3D-printed organs, manufactured organs. They are using other terminology. The term whole-organ engineering is something that is being used a lot in this context; that is why they are together.
Andrés García	I understand that, but the question is, we are going to come up with a definition, and we want it to be, not only today, but into the future. I think we should have it as general and as encompassing as possible. I understand your point, I just don't understand why we are limiting it to that.
William Wagner	We could. I think, in that case, it would be one of these where there's a multi-definition.
Joachim Kohn	Could I make an amendment to Dr. Garcia's point? If you take out, "by the recellularization and subsequent recellularization of organs," and just continue, that results in the preservation, you actually have a good definition that leaves it open by which means you achieve the end goal. The engineering of replacement organs that results in the preservation of tissue type specific matrix, and then it is just independent of the particular method.
Arthur Coury	I am assuming this is either allogeneic or xenogeneic, and I don't know if we should be specifying whether that is the case. Secondly, you could transplant a part of a liver. That you may be treated in some way. You could transplant parts of the area of a body of skin, and that is why I have had trouble with this whole organ transplant.
William Wagner	A part of the skin would not a whole organ. I would say part of a liver would not be a whole liver.

Arthur Coury	It functions as a whole liver; it is going to regenerate.
Rena Bizios	I would like to go back to what Joachim said. Did I understand your suggestion correctly of saying that this whole-organ engineering as in the engineering and obtaining whole organs by various methods? One of the methods could be 3D printing. Another method could be the decellularization-recellularization method. The third method would be microfluidics, who knows what? Is that what you meant?
Joachim Kohn	Yes.
Rena Bizios	I like that suggestion, because if we include this, but we expand a little bit more the methods which even currently have been explored, and who knows what the future will bring, because here it is only one "approach method."
Wei Sun	Also, I would like to see this definition to be more inclusive rather than to be very exclusive. I like to leave some room for organ printing, 3D printing, because that probably will represent one of the important technology for this generation here.
William Wagner	There is an edit now that I think captures what Joachim said.
Cato Laurencin	All right, why don't we vote. Let us see how controversial this is.

(d) Final Definition and Voting for "Whole Organ Engineering"

Whole Organ Engineering

The engineering of replacement organs that results in the preservation of tissue type specific matrix in a 3D architecture that closely mimics the native tissue and seeks to provide organ-specific functionality

Voting Yes	25
Voting No	20
Abstain	3
Total Votes	48
Number voting Yes or No	45
Percentage Yes Votes	55.6%

The definition achieved Provisional Consensus, having more than 50% Yes votes.

H Scaffold

(a) Possible Definitions of "Scaffold" Included in Final Program

A porous structure which serves as a substrate and guide for tissue regeneration

(b) William Wagner; Perspectives on "Scaffold" and Suggested Definition

William Wagner	Okay, related to that one. I am sure we'll have some discussion. Scaffold: a porous structure which serves as a substrate and guide for tissue regeneration.

A porous structure which serves as a substrate and guide for tissue regeneration

(c) Edited Discussion of "Scaffold"

Rena Bizios	I think we have to put porous material structure. We have to put material, whether you like material, biomaterial, whatever, but it has to be material. It is not only a structure.
William Wagner	How would it be structured if it were not a material.
Andrés García	I suggest we take out the word "porous."
Cato Laurencin	Agreement? You're agreement to that? I am shaking up heads, yes. Different ways.
Arthur Coury	I was going to say because a monolithic hydrogel containing cells has been considered a scaffold for tissue regeneration.
Deon Bezuidenhout	I think late in the session or in another session we are going to start talking about matrices, and in the minds of many of my students, these terms are often confused or used instead of one other. So I think the porous nature of this which in my eyes at least, a porous scaffold is a micron sized or macroporosity, whereas in a matrix, I understand it to be maybe to be a hydrogel, which is also porous, but just much smaller.
Deon Bezuidenhout	Maybe in two hundred Angstrom, or whatever size. I would vote for the retention of "porous."
Serena Best	Can I just put forward "3-dimensional structure?"
Xiaobing Fu	Maybe it is a tool to repair and regenerate, because repair and regeneration are quite different. So, I hope there is a separation of repair and regeneration.
Cato Laurencin	Repair and regeneration, yes. Let us talk about the 3-dimensional. I guess there are these cell sheet scaffold systems that are 2-D systems. I am not sure whether they have to be absolutely 3D.
Bikramjit Basu	I would like to add this structure with interconnected porosity.
Cato Laurencin	Interconnected porosity? We just took our porosity, you want to put in interconnected. So we decided to go without porosity.
Changsheng Liu	A scaffold is this bandwidth of material, that has structure so more than just structure.
Cato Laurencin	So what would your suggestion be?
Changsheng Liu	A kind of material, with a special structure, which serves to repair tissues or for cell growth.
Cato Laurencin	There's a blatant structure that the material should be in, included.
Changsheng Liu	Scaffold, no this scaffold is a structure, but a structure is not a scaffold.

Nicholas Peppas	Based on this definition, is the metallic mesh of a stent a scaffold?
William Wagner	It's a non-degradable scaffold.
Nicholas Peppas	But you would call it a scaffold. The mesh of the stent.
William Wagner	The stent is ...
Nicholas Peppas	I don't mean the whole stent. The mesh, just the mesh. It is a structure that serves as a substrate ...
William Wagner	But the mesh is a stent.
Nicholas Peppas	I guess what I am leaning to I would have preferred to see the word "porous structure" of a polymer or a porous structure of a biomaterial, something like that.
William Wagner	Metals can be scaffolds.
Nicholas Peppas	It may be better to start with "biomaterial with 2-dimensional structure which serves as a guide." In this way, some other aspects are covered.
William Wagner	So with the structure or biomaterial.
Nicholas Peppas	A biomaterial with 2-dimensional structure.
William Wagner	Can we call the question generally? I want to make an edit and make a vote, and try to get one more term in if we can. So, biomaterial, hands up, or structure. So first, biomaterial? Okay, well we are not asking that yet. Structure?
Cato Laurencin	Or how about "biomaterial structure?" Biomaterial structure. Very good, yes? You had a question or are you going to say the same thing?
Yunbing Wang	In fact, just now, I would like to say biomaterial structure, because that an echo to Nicholas Peppas' questions for biodegradable stents now in use especially for medical areas, people always call scaffold, people who sell them call the stent. So using "biomaterials scaffold" might be better.
Cato Laurencin	Alright, we are going to call the question when we vote. Do you have a comment to make? Go ahead. Quick comment?
Rui Reis	I think if you put "biomaterial" that does not include the cell sheet, so the question is if we want to include the cell sheet technologies into that, and then we cannot put 3-D, and we cannot put biomaterial. If we do not want it there, then it should be in some other place. But if you want to include the cell sheets, that biomaterials structure will not solve the situation.
Cato Laurencin	It was just going to get to yes with biomaterials structure. Let's vote.

(d) Final Definition and Voting for "Scaffold"

Scaffold

A biomaterial structure which serves as a substrate and guide for tissue repair and regeneration

Voting Yes	38
Voting No	9
Abstain	0
Total Votes	47
Number voting Yes or No	47
Percentage Yes Votes	80.9%

The definition achieved Consensus, having more than 75% Yes votes, with absolute number greater than 30.

(e) Further Commentary on the Definition of "Scaffold"

In the context that David Williams was given the authority to make minor grammatical alterations, a slightly better wording is as follows; it is this which is confirmed to have consensus:

Scaffold

A biomaterial structure that serves as a substrate and guide for tissue repair and regeneration

I Template

(a) Possible Definitions of "Template" Included in Final Program

Biomaterials-based construct of defined size, chemistry and architecture that controls the delivery of molecular and mechanical signals to target cells in tissue engineering processes[3]

(b) William Wagner; Perspectives on "Template" and Suggested Definition

William Wagner   Why don't we go with template? This should keep us going. "Biomaterials-based construct of defined size, chemistry, and architecture that controls the delivery of molecular, mechanical signals to target cells and tissue engineering processes."

(c) Edited Discussion of "Template"

Nicholas Peppas   The term is absolutely perfect when one looks at tissue engineering. I have no problem with it. But as you know in the last 10 years, many of us are using the term "template" in molecular imprinting, in putting specific structures inside a polymer to create a new advanced structure for recognition purposes.

Nicolas Peppas

---

[3] Williams DF, The biomaterials conundrum in tissue engineering, *Tissue Engineering*, Part A, 2014;20:1129-31.

	It is a minor point, but it is an area that is expanding, including our own group. This is a little bit confusing. People who work with templates and molecular imprinting will see this and say: "Well, this is not the same."
Cato Laurencin	Alright. David?
David Williams	I understand what you are saying there. Maybe it's one area where the same word is used very correctly into a different context, and I think we have to allow for that. The reason why I have for several years now referred to templates as an alternative to scaffolds is this. People use scaffold, that's fine, but scaffold is a very, very limited concept. If you think of a scaffold as normally on the outside of a building, when you are putting a building up, the scaffolds are then taken down having played no role whatsoever in the actual construction of the building. It is just a tool.
Cate Laurencin	Other comments? I think itis a great definition.
John Brash	Yes, can we now just call this a tissue template? To take care of Nick's comment. And there are other kinds of template, which are still in the biomaterials sphere, such as molecular imprinting, for example. This is a tissue template, that is what it is really saying. I think in that definition.
Cato Laurencin	David, do you have a preference on that?
David Williams	Yes, I understand what John is saying. "Tissue template" sounds a bit clumsy to me. I would much rather just "template." And then we could have two different definitions or two different definitions. I am not comfortable with "tissue template." It implies a template made of tissue, for example.
Cato Laurencin	Yes, I think parenthetically, we use the term "scaffold," but I know the term "scaffold" is used in lots of other areas of medicine, but we understand it in the biomaterials world, where at least right now we are thinking about it now that way.
Rena Bizios	So perhaps to resolve this particular situation is to target cells for various biomedical applications. You can find better words there, such as "tissue engineering," and that leaves it open to some other applications, where there is tissue engineering or something else.
Cato Laurencin	I think we have tissue engineering processes. Right now, it says that. Is that . . .
Rena Bizios	Yes, saying to put it in biomedical or something more general in terms, such as tissue engineering, because then it opens it up for other applications that Nicholas mentioned. That is all I am saying. I didn't say to include tissue engineering to make it biomedical, or broader term, and then an example will be tissue engineering.
Cato Laurencin	Nick is saying that the definition, if it was for these other areas, actually is not . . . this isn't a definition at all.

Nicholas Peppas	An objection; we can proceed with tissue engineering, it is very well done. Forget molecular imprinting, we can discuss it some other time.
Maria J. Vincent	Right now, to include both, if we act like a sentence, saying that that controls the macro or microstructure on the delivery of the molecular, because what the molecular imprinting does, is really modifying the macro or microstructure of the polymer itself. The template. So maybe we can include it. I don't know.
David Williams	I understand what you are saying, but I think that does tend to confuse it, if we tried to put them together into one definition.
David Williams	As Nick said, forget molecular imprinting for a moment.
Cato Laurencin	Alright.
Hua Ai	So for template source, templates are also used for other systems. To load drugs in. As other colleagues in the field in nanotechnology, they all use templates for drug theory applications. I think maybe it is not only for tissue engineering.
Cato Laurencin	So, I guess this is template ... is applied to tissue engineering.
Joachim Kohn	Then I just want to put everyone at ease, because when you look at the definition of the word "cell," it can be a prison cell, a terrorist cell, a cellphone, a mammalian cell, and it is understood that the same word has different meanings.
Cato Laurencin	We are not going to find that, no matter what you want.
Joachim Kohn	Yes, in different fields. So I agree with David actually. This is understood to be actually, in our field, and that is our definition. And obviously in other fields they do different things, and so we don't really need to concern ourselves about that.
Cato Laurencin	Alright.
Joachim Kohn	Let's keep it clean and simple.

(d) Final Definition and Voting for "Template"

Template

Biomaterials-based construct of defined size, chemistry and architecture that controls the delivery of molecular and mechanical signals to target cells in tissue engineering processes

Voting Yes	32
Voting No	14
Abstain	1
Total Votes	47
Number voting Yes or No	46
Percentage Yes Votes	69.5%

The definition achieved Provisional Consensus, having more than 50% Yes votes.

J Immunoisolation

(a) Possible Definitions of "Immunoisolation" Included in Final Program

An immunological strategy in which non-self antigens that are present on an allograft or xenograft are prevented from coming into contact with the host immune system

(b) William Wagner; Perspectives on "Immunoisolation" and Suggested Definition

William Wagner	Immunoisolation, another term used all the time, immunoisolation using devices and encapsulation, "an immunological strategy in which non-self antigens that are present on an allograft or xenograft are prevented from coming into contact with the host immune system."

(c) Edited Discussion of "Immunoisolation"

Elizabeth Cosgriff-H	I would just possibly make the allograft and xenograft broader and to be able to include cells in that. The allograft is tissue, as opposed to just cells. And maybe take out the immunological strategy.
William Wagner	I think cells are considered a graft.
Elizabeth Cosgriff-H	Okay.
Cato Laurencin	It would be part of a graft, yes. Other comments?
Rena Bizios	That is fine, but I think we should consider emphasizing more than just the concept. It is a response, and most likely it is an adverse response, so is there a suggestion of expanding that and replacing it with something that is a little more to the point.
Cato Laurencin	Suggestion? What do you think.
Rena Bizios	For me it is not only context. Yes, we have to come to context, but then show all kinds of adverse responses. How to phrase that? Right now I cannot suggest it.
Cato Laurencin	So you are saying to prevent it from having interactions with the host immune system.
Andres Garcia	Yes, two points. Most of those strategies are not specific to non-self antigens, while get rid of non-self, and the current technology of any of this immunoisolation technologies, what they are really preventing is direct contact with the host immune system. I don't know if we want to put direct contact with immune system.
William Wagner	Yes, I think non-self is redundant with antigenic, it's … You are saying what now for the cells?
Andrés García	I think we have to be specific to say that this strategy, what they prevent is direct contact and it is really cellular whole system.
William Wagner	So you want to add direct contact?

Andrés García	I would argue that we have to add direct there.
William Wagner	Why do you need direct as opposed to contact?
Andrés García	Because none of the strategies prevents a shed antigen to get out … If you think of an islet encapsulation, right? The islet can still shed antigens that get out and interact with the host system through one indirect pathway.
Cato Laurencin	Alright, but that would be a good strategy if that is what you need in terms of immunoisolation.
Andrés García	That is what you need but nobody has done that.
Laura Poole-Warren	My question was, are they all immunological strategies? Or are they actually just strategies? Because some of them are based on size exclusion, et cetera. So it is not necessarily an immunological strategy, so I would perhaps suggest removing the second word.
William Wagner	Any opposition to that?
Andrés García	I think it's a good point.
Cato Laurencin	It is a good point. Last contribution? Other comments? We are ready to vote? Okay. Vote one for yes, two for no. Alright. Our verdict?
Cato Laurencin	Alright, very good, thank you.

(d) Final Definition and Voting for "Immunoisolation"

Immunoisolation

A strategy in which antigens that are present on an allograft or xenograft are prevented from coming into direct contact with the host immune system

Voting Yes	43
Voting No	3
Abstain	2
Total Votes	48
Number voting Yes or No	46
Percentage Yes Votes	93.5%

The definition achieved Consensus, having more than 75% Yes votes, with absolute number greater than 30.

K Other Regenerative Medicine-Related Terms: No Voting, With or Without Discussion

A number of other terms were scheduled for discussion and voting during Session III but time allowed for only limited discussion and no votes were taken. The definitions proposed by the Plenary Speaker are included here for completeness.

Cell Therapy

The process of introducing new cells into a tissue in order to treat disease; *Williams DF, Essential Biomaterials Science, Cambridge University Press, 2014*

Self-Assembly

1. The autonomous organization of components into patterns or structures without human intervention[4]
2. The autonomous organization of components into patterns or structures without management from outside sources

Tissue Integration

The functional incorporation of engineered tissue into a host

Tissue Equivalent

A product that is intended to replace or augment natural tissue and which has properties that are analogous to those of that tissue

Provisional Matrix

A loosely organized ECM that is developed at the site of tissue injury that is characterized by fibrin and other components of the hemostatic system

[4] *Whitesides GM & Grzybowski B, Self-assembly at all scales, Science 2002;295:2418.*

VII

Biomaterial-based devices

Discussed in Session IV

Session IV Plenary Presentation: *Jiang Chang*
Session IV Moderator: *Arthur Coury*
Session III Reporter: *Keith McLean*

A Implant

(a) Possible Definitions of "Implant" Included in Final Program

Implant (synonymous with Implantable Device)
A medical device made from one or more biomaterials that is intentionally placed within the body, either totally or partially buried beneath an epithelial surface; *Definition that achieved consensus in Chester, 1986*

(b) Jiang Chang; Perspectives on "Implant" and Suggested Definition

Jiang Chang	The first term we choose is implant because we think it is really important for our session. So implant is actually, it reached a consensus 30 years ago, so an implant is "a medical device made from one or more biomaterials that is intentionally placed within the body, either totally or partially buried beneath the epithelial surface." So I let you start a discussion.

(c) Edited Discussion of "Implant"

Ruggero Bettini	Yes. I have a concern with respect to the definition, to the limitation of the definition to a medical device. In my vision, an implant can be also a medicinal product.
Nicholas Peppas	I can see what Ruggero says. It could be medicinal. But I have another question. I just don't like this word "buried" or "partially buried." Can we find another word?
Arthur Coury	Thank you. I guess. Yes. "placed"? - is that a better word?

Laura Poole-Warren	You could just remove "buried."
Arthur Coury	Okay.
Laura Poole-Warren	Placed within the body either totally or partially.
Arthur Coury	Does that change of words, that seems to be okay for us to proceed? We'll try to make changes along the way as we can.
Rena Bizios	I have a question. Why so much emphasis, exclusive emphasis, on epithelial surfaces? I mean, implants can be inside all sorts of other tissues. They are not necessarily epithelial containing surfaces or tissues, in my opinion.
Arthur Coury	I think the epithelium is the outside layer of all of the tissue, and if it's an implant, you have to penetrate that. So that's what you're doing. You're going under it.
Rena Bizios	But without specifying if it is buried, it is inside already. It's not just underneath. It is part of inside tissues. I have a feeling I am proposing that we have to consider modifying that particular statement to be a little bit more inclusive of all kinds of tissues.
Bikramjit Basu	So if when it is said that it is intentionally placed within the body, then I think that body beneath an epithelial tissue may not be necessary.
Bikramjit Basu	The other thing that is missing in this definition is that to restore the functionality, for example, hip implant, so it is, it will restore the functionality of the hip joint. Similarly knee implants will restore the function of the knee joints. Restoring the functionality that can be included in this definition.
Arthur Coury	Comments on that? I think that limits it maybe beyond what it should be limited. Because sometimes you want to decrease functionality.
David Williams	Art, can I just answer that? I understand what you mean by functionality, but there are some soft tissue implants which are there simply to change shape, and that's not necessarily function.
David Williams	I also understand what Laura is saying. You could just have it in the body, either totally or partially, period.
Arthur Coury	Yes. I think that's good. You are defining an implant that way, that it goes partially or completely under an epithelial surface.
Rena Bizios	It is either; you place it within the body among tissues. We do not have to specify epithelial surfaces or anything else. That is really restrictive in my mind.
Mário Barbosa	This is really a naïve question. Is ear piercing an implant according to this definition? An ear piercing. Is it an implant? Yes? It would be.
David Williams	No, no, no. It's not.
Mário Barbosa	No? Yes or no?

David Williams	It is not a medical device.
Yunbing Wang	How about remove "intentionally" and the "buried"? These two words.
Yunbing Wang	Just say "a medical device made from one or more biomaterials that is placed within the body either totally or partially, beneath an epithelial surface."
Arthur Coury	Good. That sounds good. Get rid of those two words. Yes?
Nicholas Peppas	I don't know if you want to include that, but it relates to what Professor Bizios said. Is an intraocular lens an implant? That is in the epithelium, and it is buried or hidden or placed under. Do you want that?
Arthur Coury	I definitely feel that it's an implant.
Jiang Chang	I don't think that.
Hua Ai	Yes. I think so.
Arthur Coury	And it is behind an epithelium, of course.
Rena Bizios	Should we include here some as regarding the time into, the length of time that these things are going to be inside the body? Are they permanently or implanted for the life span of the recipient, or is it not a necessary part of this definition, the time aspect?
Arthur Coury	I think I would have that as a separate definition, as a chronic or subchronic or acute implant. But I don't think we need to get into that with this broad definition.
David Williams	The word "intentionally" has been removed. That was there for a reason. For example, if a surgeon is operating inside a patient and working with a medical device which is a retractor and accidentally leaves it behind, that is not going to be an implant. That is a real problem. That was really why "intentionally" was there.
Arthur Coury	That's right. I would restore "intentional." Put it back in.
Xingdong Zhang	Also I think the "intentionally" cannot be removed because we list the definition is for implant. The intention can't be removed.
Iulian Antoniac	I think a sentence about the clinical benefit must be added to this definition. Because the implant must have a clinical benefit, in my opinion, and because also surgical instruments complete this definition.
Arthur Coury	That is either implied or it needs to be stated. What do we think?
Kai Zhang	I was going to comment on this. I don't know what the story behind the phrase "beneath the epithelial surface," was. We seem to have a lot of discussion on this. But I just suggest we can probably remove it totally or partially, just between the intentionally placed. So it will be "a medical device made from one or more biomaterials that has intentionally, either totally or partially, been placed within the body."

Kai Zhang	But also try to separate implant from surgical instruments. Those will also be intentionally placed within the body during the surgery, so those are not implants. We know that.
Arthur Coury	And the one thing is that there are some devices now that go in internally through, you know, that you swallow, for example, into the stomach, and I do like epithelial, getting under an epithelial surface. David? What do you think? You agree?
David Williams	I'm fairly ambivalent about that. I understand what you're saying, but to me, I am fine either way on that one.
Carl Simon	The term medical device would exclude things with biological effects, like a drug eluting stent would not be an implant any longer. And then a tissue engineered-product would not be an implant.
Arthur Coury	Not at all. The drug eluting stent is a medical device.
Carl Simon	But doesn't that have biological effect?
Arthur Coury	Yes.
Carl Simon	Because the definition of medical device, as far as I know, does not primarily work by effecting a chemical change in the body.
Arthur Coury	If it primarily, and a stent doesn't. That is still defined as a device. So does a drug eluting pacemaker lead. Because its main effect is electrical sensing and stimulating. Here, the main effect in a stent is mechanical, keeping the blood vessel open with or without a drug.
Carl Simon	Well, would it have the same meaning if you just removed the word "medical," because if you just said a device, then it would lose the regulatory aspect and it would include any type of device that was implanted. Or do you really want to say that it has to be a medical device?
Jiang Chang	Yeah. I think, I agree. Personally, I think we can remove the "medical." Just say a device.
Carl Simon	Because, again, by the definition that David had put forth for a medical device, even though we did not vote on it, a lot of things that we think of as implants would not be included if you make it specific to medical device.
David Williams	If you take out the word "medical," then many other things come into the definition, which we do not want.
Carl Simon	True.
David Williams	I do not think that is what we're asking.
Carl Simon	Is there another word we can put there? A therapeutic device.
Arthur Coury	It is a medical device.
Rena Bizios	David said that if we remove medical device we have to put a statement that Dr. Park had suggested about what is the reason?
Carl Simon	What about a therapeutic device?

Rena Bizios	Because if it is a medical application or something like that, the medical device there does not necessitate the extra statement at the end.
Arthur Coury	And you could have an implant that is totally diagnostic.
David Williams	Or cosmetic.
Arthur Coury	Or cosmetic. I would stick with medical device myself.
Timmie Topoleski	I wanted to go back to what I think Professor Antoniac said. What in this definition would exclude something like a scalpel used during surgery? It's a medical device. It's intentionally placed within the body, and partially beneath an epithelium. But it is not intended to stay there.
Arthur Coury	Yes. Intended for medical benefit or something like that? Could be diagnostic, therapeutic. It could even be delivering a drug.
Rena Bizios	The therapeutic benefit is there for all of the above. The thing that makes Topoleski's comment relevant to me is the aspect of time. That is a very temporary use of the device coming in contact with physiological tissues. An implant that goes as a hip prosthesis or a cardiovascular graft, it's a totally different story because it is going to be in the body permanently or for the duration of the life of the recipient. I think that is what Tim is trying to bring to our attention.
Arthur Coury	Sometimes we implant a catheter for a few hours, twelve hours, sixteen hours.
Arthur Coury	But it's still an implant, so look at this … If we want it to say for beneficial medical purposes, that would be good. Would you go with that? You could put that in. And I do think we have to start moving on. I thought this one would be a quick one.
Elizabeth Cosgriff-H	No, I feel like that circumvents a lot of the cosmetic things that may not have clear medical benefit.
Arthur Coury	But those are not medical devices?
Elizabeth Cosgriff-H	Yes, they are.
Arthur Coury	Oh, then it has a beneficial medical purpose. I thought you meant something like an injection or something.
William Wagner	I think a medical device, there are no medical devices that are out there that are not intended to provide some kind of benefit. I think the argument about, it needs to say more than that, I think we're wordsmithing the heck out of something that was pretty good to begin with.
Arthur Coury	No. I think David's mention of it, of an unintentional implant. That, that was implied.
Kai Zhang	Again, I still couldn't tell an implant from a surgical instrument from this definition.

Cato Laurencin	They could be the same. If you ever fracture a bone and you use a drill and you drill a screw, that drill bit, that drill bit is used as an implant. Part of it is an implant. You throw it away. If you have a knife, a scalpel, the, I mean, most scalpel blades you use, that's actually charged as an implant.
Kai Zhang	I always saw those as surgical instruments. And it can be throw away.
Ling Qin	Just ask question on the epithelial, means skin, if it is, it is more popular.
Arthur Coury	It could be your soft palate, it could be your nasal cartilage, as epithelia.
Ling Qin	Otherwise, people think a really more, for known medical, people among, non-biological people would be confused with it. If just about, I say place the, partially or totally within the body could be easier.
Rena Bizios	May I make a suggestion regarding the comments that were made, putting at the end, after surface, for various periods of time. And that brings all kinds of aspects which are pertinent to all of these little things.
Arthur Coury	For that, but it is always for various periods of time, I think. You would have to state acute, sub-acute or chronic.
Rena Bizios	It is going to be for long periods of time or something like that.
Arthur Coury	But it doesn't have to be acute implant.
Rena Bizios	It doesn't.
Andrés García	So, I am still concerned by the point that Carl raised about a medical device and somebody reading that strictly from a regulatory standpoint. Could we add, or combination device? Just something to move away or, that is not moving away from the regulatory decision, but at least expanding the scope of what the implant could be.
Carl Simon	But we could try to avoid the, the use of the word device and try to go back to a medical purpose, so something made from one or more biomaterials that is intentionally placed within the body for medical purposes. Something general like that.
Joachim Kohn	Yes. I endorse this because I was thinking about, for instance, the vaginal rings that are inserted for contraceptive purposes. Most women would think of it as an implant. It is inserted but not necessarily under an epithelial layer. It is actually inside an epithelial surface. Right? And so this definition is really, on first sight I understand. It is very trivial actually, but when you think about it, it gets complicated. So would you think a vaginal ring for contraceptive purposes is an implant?
Arthur Coury	Elizabeth, what would you call it.
Elizabeth Cosgriff-H	I would not, but I don't know what I would call it.

Arthur Coury	There's also the scleral buckle that's around the outside of the eyeball, and it generates fibrous capsules and everything, and some people call it an exoplant, but I wouldn't call it a vaginal ring an exoplant.
Carl Simon	So, I'm on the FDA website, and they don't make the exclusion that I can see about the biological effect. Implant is a device that is placed into a surgically or naturally formed cavity of the human body and is intended to remain there for a period of 30 days or more in order to protect the public health. Blah, blah, blah. So I don't know. You had that bit in there about not being a pharmacological factor, so I don't know. Maybe that doesn't apply. So maybe medical device is okay. I assumed you got your definition from the FDA or another regulatory agency.
Arthur Coury	We could go on and on and on. I would feel maybe we should drop, then, the epithelial penetration part of it. And that would be in line with the FDA. They're not specifying whether it is a natural cavity or a non-natural cavity.
Kai Zhang	I will point out I think the FDA made a good point on the 30 days or longer. There's a time period there. I mean, I just could not tell the surgical instrument and the catheter as implants.
Arthur Coury	I feel strongly that the FDA use the terms chronic or subacute, subchronic, subacute, acute, and chronic, and all of those can refer to implants. I think I am getting nods. So. Excuse me.
Jiang Chang	I am just thinking because I heard the comments that maybe we can remove the beneath an epithelial surface. Someone suggested. Personally, I think that that should be okay.
Arthur Coury	So we vote on this when Professor Chang removes that last part. Okay. Are we okay? Are we ready to vote?

(d) Final Definition and Voting for "Implant"

Implant

A medical device made from one or more biomaterials that is intentionally placed, either totally or partially, within the body

Voting Yes	37
Voting No	7
Abstain	0
Total Votes	44
Number voting Yes or No	44
Percentage Yes Votes	84.1%

The definition achieved Consensus, having more than 75% Yes votes, with absolute number greater than 30.

B Percutaneous and Transcutaneous

(a) Possible Definitions of "Percutaneous and Transcutaneous" Included in Final Program

Percutaneous: Taking place through the skin, involving disruption of the skin. Transcutaneous: Passing through the intact skin. *Note "per" and "trans" both could mean "through" or "across." Convention and usage now determines that with respect to skin, "per" implies that passage through the skin involves some degree of physical penetration whereas "trans" implies the skin remains intact*

(b) Jiang Chang; Perspectives on "Percutaneous and Transcutaneous" and Suggested Definition

Jiang Chang	So now we move to the next. Here we have two, which are similar. One is "percutaneous," which means taking place through the skin involving disruption of the skin. The other is "transcutaneous," penetrating, entering or passing through the intact skin. Both are actually from David's suggestion.
Jiang Chang	Okay, please note that "per" and "trans" both could mean through or across. And convention and usage now determines that with respect to skin. "Per" implies that passage through the skin involves some degree of physical penetration, whereas "trans" implies the skin remains intact.

(c) Edited Discussion of "Percutaneous and Transcutaneous"

Arthur Coury	So the way that we could approach this one is to have the two definitions with a caveat. Does that sound like a reasonable way to do it, David?
David Williams	When I looked at this, as the note says, as far as I could see, a very clear definition in the literature of the difference between "per" and "trans" as given there. For example, transdermal delivery of drugs compared to a percutaneous interventional device in cardiology. So I think they are different. I would rather see two definitions myself. The text will show that difference.
Arthur Coury	That's the way I teach my courses, that "trans" means across, intact skin, and "per" means through the skin. But I do think that keeping in line with good English language, we should have that caveat statement. Are there any comments, please?

Editor's Note: There were no comments.

(d) Final Definitions and Voting, taken together, for "Percutaneous" and "Transcutaneous"

Percutaneous

Taking place through the skin, involving disruption of the skin

Transcutaneous
Penetrating, entering or passing through the intact skin

Voting Yes	42
Voting No	0
Abstain	0
Total Votes	42
Number voting Yes or No	42
Percentage Yes Votes	100%

The definition achieved Consensus, having more than 75% Yes votes, with absolute number greater than 30.

C Prosthesis

(a) Possible Definitions of "Prosthesis" Included in Final Program

Device that replaces or supports a limb, organ or tissue of a body

(b) Jiang Chang; Perspectives on "Prosthesis" and Suggested Definition

Jiang Chang   The next term is "prosthesis," which is being defined in Professor Williams's dictionary, which means a device that replaces a limb, organ or tissue of a body. But we also have some discussion and would like to suggest a minor revision, which means not only replaces, but it is also possible to support. So the suggestion is device that replaces or supports a limb, organ or tissue of a body.

(c) Edited Discussion of "Prosthesis"

David Williams   Could I comment on that one? The second, the new suggestion there, to me that would include an orthosis, which is an external structured support, for example for a leg which is deficient, and that is not replacing it. It is supporting, and to me that is not a prosthesis.

Arthur Coury   Well let us discuss that. To me it is, but let us have expert opinions on this. It is a tough one if you haven't thought so much about it.

David Williams   I think there is an important difference. Functionally these are very different. If you are talking about, for example, a lower limb, artificial lower limb, functionality is very different to having a leg which is still intact and then you put some carbon fiber structure around it to help movement, that is the orthosis. Functionally and structurally that is very different.

Arthur Coury	I see what you mean. What are dental braces? Aren't those prosthetic devices? Yes, Professor Bizios bring some logic to us here.
Rena Bizios	I don't give the answer to your question or statement, but because the topic of this session is implantable, my suggestion is to make the device implantable, or implanted devices that replace and support the limb. It is not an outside placement to support the limb. It would make it "implanted devices," or "implantable," whatever the appropriate word there is, "which replace or support a limb, organ or tissue of body."
Jiang Chang	Okay, I support actually if we just look at logistics, support a limb might be okay, but to support an organ or tissue makes no sense. So original definition might be more applicable.
Arthur Coury	I think tissues are everything in the body, you know. From blood to bones, to skin to soft tissue, so it is very general, but I don't think I would remove that, because there could be situations where you would be dealing with soft tissue. David?
David Williams	I still think there is a difference. For example, up until very recently one of the most widely used prostheses were dental prostheses, which are placed in the mouth. They are not supporting the mouth, they are there to replace teeth and part the palate, and that is a classic prosthesis. I still think that we should not talk about supporting it.
Elizabeth Cosgriff-H	Do we add in "replaces the function of a limb, organ or tissue?" To create that functional aspect?
Arthur Coury	Yes it would be. You know a cast on the leg would work, but I have to defer to David, who has more expertise in this. So I would suggest that we remove this. The word, or "supports." Is there anybody that objects to that? Anybody object to that removal?
John Ramshaw	David, I don't know the surgery, but in pelvic organ prolapse, is the mesh that is put in there, put in to support the tissues, and therefore should "supports" stay into that option?
David Williams	Yes, the mesh is there to support, but I do not know anywhere that would be described as a prosthesis. It is not a prosthesis. A mesh is there to facilitate healing, while supporting the tissue.
John Ramshaw	Okay, fine.
Arthur Coury	And so now we are suggesting that we remove "or supports."
Timmie Topoleski	What about something like a left ventricular assist device, which is helping function, and it is supporting a partially functioning part of the body? Another I was wondering is, I know maybe David, you don't like this in a definition, but using a phrase in contrast to a prosthetic or orthotic.
David Williams	You are correct, I do not like it.

Timmie Topoleski	Sorry.
Cato Laurencin	I am just a bone doctor, but when we think about prostheses we think about replacing a body part, not replacing a tissue.
Arthur Coury	But replacing, not just replacing versus supporting, we are completely replacing.
Cato Laurencin	But support, in some cases, you can have a prosthesis that, say a partial replacement that augments something, but it's really- we learn that prostheses help actually replace things. Orthoses actually help things work. That is the difference between the two.
David Williams	Can I come back on the left ventricular assist device? I do not believe that is a prosthesis, because it is not replacing, physically replacing the ventricle. It is there to support the function. We would not call that a prosthesis at all.
Arthur Coury	I would tend to, Cato, to lean to more of the broad definition because of things we are not thinking of as including now, or in the future. What would be your suggested change?
Rena Bizios	Along those lines, device that replaces a part of the body, such as a limb. I like the part of the body replacement, Cato. So, "such as a limb," gives an example.
Arthur Coury	Can we say "a body part?" And we don't like the use of examples. How about that?
Cato Laurencin	"A body part" is fine.
Nicholas Peppas	You have two Greeks in the audience, who tell you that prosthesis, in Greek, prosthesis means "addition." And of course, it can be a replacement. Addition or replacement, okay? Prosthesis is addition, so.
Arthur Coury	Of a body part.?
Carl Simon	So again, I'm on the FDA website, and they do use the word "support." "...or provide support to organs and tissues," when they describe it, just putting that out there. But they also use "replace." So, they include both, "support" and "replace."
Arthur Coury	So, let's have a vote on both definitions. How's that? I think that maybe the best way to do it. So put both of them down. One is just "replace," and one is "replace or support," but I like "a body part."
Arthur Coury	So first thing we're going to vote on is the first definition, because we spent a lot of time removing that word. And then we are going to vote on the second.
Arthur Coury	Rena?
Rena Bizios	What is the body part?
Jiang Chang	So change to "the body part," so it is the limb only?
Arthur Coury	But they are different, because one adds that really important term, "or supports." Yes, let us replace the enumeration by "a body part."

Carl Simon	Maybe instead of "support," if people don't like "support" because they think of a physical support, it could be "assists," or "assists with the function of a limb, organ or tissue."
Arthur Coury	What does the FDA use, though? Because I would not want to vary too far from that.
Carl Simon	"Medical implants are devices or tissues that are placed inside or on the surface of the body. Many implants are prosthetics intended to replace missing body parts. Other implants deliver medication, monitor body functions, or provide support to organs or tissues. Some implants are made from skin, bone or other body tissues. Others are made from metal, plastic, ceramic or other tissues."
Arthur Coury	So I think again, let us just vote on these two, and we will vote on number one first. And actually we will vote on number two anyhow, but let us see. This is weird, but let's try it. We are voting on the top definition.
Timmie Topoleski	Or you could just vote on whether to include the term "or supports" and have one vote.
Arthur Coury	Okay. I like that. Okay so, here is the way we are do it. If you like the use of the words "or supports," then you vote one. No, you put the number one down, that's what I meant, I didn't say vote on. Alright, we're just going to vote once if we like that, "or supports," then we are going with it. If we don't, then we'll vote on the second, without "or supports," okay?
Arthur Coury	So first, look at the top definition. Look at the top definition first, and if you like that- yes, remove "or supports" from the bottom. We are voting for the top one first, we shouldn't even be showing the second. Vote one if you like the top. Vote one if you like the top definition. Ready, set, go. With the word "support."
William Wagner	Art the only issue with doing this is if we each have our own favorite definition, then neither of them may pass.
Arthur Coury	That is right.
William Wagner	But if you just put one of them up there, then we might still vote for that one. Because right now I am going to vote "no" on the first one and "yes" on the second one, because I like the second one. See what I am saying? So you might just want to pick your favorite one as plenary and have us vote on that.
Arthur Coury	Okay. Because it is not making it.
Jiang Chang	I think at any rate we change to "body parts," yes?
Arthur Coury	Yes. That is a body part. So clearly that one didn't make it, and I am not sure the next one will make it, but let us vote on that. Does everybody have numbers down that are needed?
Carl Simon	Art you may want to do a revote, because they got switched halfway through the voting. What I voted for isn't up there anymore. Sorry, it's changed.

Arthur Coury	Okay? I am sorry, I apologize, We are going to vote for this one again. If you would like that, vote one, if you don't, two, if you want to abstain, vote three.

(d) Final Definitions and Voting for "Prosthesis"

First Vote

Prosthesis

Device that replaces or supports a body part

Voting Yes	34
Voting No	13
Abstain	0
Total Votes	47
Number voting Yes or No	47
Percentage Yes Votes	72.3%

The definition achieved Provisional Consensus, having more than 50% Yes votes.

Second Vote

Prosthesis

Device that replaces a body part

Voting Yes	25
Voting No	20
Abstain	0
Total Votes	45
Number voting Yes or No	45
Percentage Yes Votes	55.5%

The definition achieved Provisional Consensus, having more than 50% Yes votes.

(e) Further Commentary on the Definition of "Prosthesis"

In the context that David Williams was given the authority to make minor grammatical alterations, a few suggestions are made. Neither definition achieved consensus and so it is appropriate to consider why this was so, especially as the term has long-standing usage. There are several possibilities, two concerning the actual words in the definitions and one concerned with some confusion about the sequential nature of the voting procedure. With respect to the wording, the two apparently contentious issues were the use of "support" and the use of "body part." The group appeared to be divided on these two points. As the discussion about orthoses showed, there was disquiet over the potentially broad interpretation of "support," taking the definition outside of the conventional meaning. Several alternatives were suggested but none appeared popular. On reflection, one word that could well fit into the spirit of the concept of "support" without the very wide and varied implications of support, would be "augment." With respect to "body part," there are, in some parts of the world, rather negative associations with the phrase. It is suggested that "body part" is replaced by "parts of the body." Thus, a revised definition could be:

Prosthesis

Device that replaces or augments a part of the body

This alternative was presented to the delegates after the conference.

D Bioprosthesis

(a) Possible Definitions of "Bioprosthesis" Included in Final Program

Implantable prosthesis that consists totally or substantially of non-viable, treated, donor tissue, *Definition that achieved consensus in Chester 1986*

(b) Jiang Chang; Perspectives on "Bioprosthesis" and Suggested Definition

Jiang Chang	The next is "bioprosthesis," which is an implantable prosthesis that consists totally or substantially of non-viable, treated donor tissue, which is actually defined in Professor Williams's dictionary. But we also made the suggestions that we think "non-viable treated" may not be necessary. So the suggestion say "implantable prosthesis that consist totally and substantially of donor tissue."

(c) Edited Discussion of "Bioprosthesis"

Arthur Coury	David and I have been trying to avoid whether a material or something that does not contain cells is viable or not viable. If you have a matrix with all of the factors in it that responds to the environment, and induces cells to do something even though there are no cells on it, when is that tissue non-viable? Some people would say, when it doesn't contain cells. And I have chosen in my definitions of biomaterials, to avoid whether something is viable or not if it doesn't contain cells. I think that is a basis for discussion here.
Andrés García	Art, if we adopt the red definition, that means a kidney transplant is a prosthesis?
Arthur Coury	Yes.
Andrés García	Right? And is that what we want to mean by "bioprosthesis?"
Arthur Coury	That is a really good point, I do not know what to say. David?
David Williams	I think Andres is absolutely correct. That takes us down a route where we don't want to be. Art, I understand your concern about

non-viable, and when we initially discussed that many years ago, I think that was perfectly valid. But as we said before, "bioprosthesis" really does refer to tissue, typically derived from a xenogeneic source, which is treated, not to keep it viable and biologically active, but to use it as an implanted medical device, and that is the difficulty I have got with the red part there. You may want to take out "nonviable." "Substantially treated donor tissue" may be sufficient.

Arthur Coury	I was going to suggest taking out the word "treated,"
Arthur Coury	Is this something worthy of voting on right now? If you take out the word "nonviable" and leave the word "treated" in? I am okay with that, honestly. We are ready to vote it looks like, so let's please vote on this.
David Williams	Let's be clear. It's the first one, taking out the term "nonviable"
Arthur Coury	Take the word "nonviable" out, please. And then get rid of the second definition. Thanks, I should look there, rather than at you. Are you ready to vote, now?
Iulian Antoniac	For example, in the case of cardiovascular implants, could this "bioprosthesis" also be from animal tissue. I think that it is important to be mentioned.
Arthur Coury	In the case of animal tissue?
Iulian Antoniac	In a heart valve
Arthur Coury	Yes, I think that is what he means, right? Is that what you mean.
Iulian Antoniac	My suggestion is regarding donor tissue, tissue to replace from human or animal tissue.
Arthur Coury	Okay. If we want to include both human and animal tissue, I think we can, because really we do treat, sometimes we treat allogeneic tissue. If you want to put that in, I see no major objection. You mean both, right?
David Williams	Again that is moving away from what we conventionally talk about, and have for 30 or 40 years on bioprosthesis, which I think is correct. Otherwise, we're going down the route of a graft, which I do not think we ought to be.
Jiang Chang	So, yes this changes- okay.
William Wagner	I think "treated" is much too vague. You could treat it with antibiotic solution, and it would be an allograft. I think the "nonviable" made sense. It indicates that you have changed it in a way that it is no longer a transplant. It is no longer a viable organ. Even there are other things you may do, and as organs are preserved for longer periods of time outside the body, they are going to be subjected to more and more treatment, and that treatment is not discriminated in this definition.

Joachim Kohn	I would like to endorse what Bill Wagner said. The "nonviable" I think is really important. As some of you know, I've been leading a transplant program with face transplants and hand transplants, and we do not want to confuse the issue between viable body part transplantation and the concept of viable stasis. It is not the treating that makes the difference, it is really the fact that in the bioprosthesis there is no viable tissue anymore. Even if it was originally derived from some viable tissue.
Arthur Coury	So the human part of it evades me. I know with other transplants, there are other words, generally tissue that's not made nonviable, but what if we, you know David and I, and maybe we don't totally agree, but when is tissue nonviable?
Joachim Kohn	I think there is some confusion here. When you take a liver transplant, you can actually transport it from the Antarctica over three days to wherever you want to have it.
Arthur Coury	Right.
Joachim Kohn	And during that time it's significantly treated, but the cells are metabolically active by the time it is being put into the donor. "Bioprosthesis," in my opinion, is some kind of a source of material, which is treated to such an extent that the cells are no longer metabolically active. And that is the definition of nonviable.
Arthur Coury	It could be human tissue, then?
Joachim Kohn	Of course, it is independent of the source of this tissue.
Arthur Coury	Okay.
Joachim Kohn	But the metabolic activity of the cells is no longer there.
Arthur Coury	The cells are no longer there, but-
Joachim Kohn	Even the cells can be there.
Arthur Coury	I think I defer to the expertise of everybody here, and we could put "nonviable" back. Deon, you're ready to say something I think.
Deon Bezuidenhout	One example the way these are used is a cryopreserved donor graft. So that is human tissue that is frozen, and the cells are no longer living. So that isn't viable.
Arthur Coury	And this brings up the question, is it viable or not? If the cells are no longer living, but you put it in and-
Joachim Kohn	You know the definition of viable is really easy. You isolate a cell population out of the implant, and put them in tissue pouch and if they still grow, they are viable.
Arthur Coury	I have avoided whether the matrix is viable, but I defer.
Joachim Kohn	A matrix is not viable. A matrix is not defined by viability. The matrix, I meant the ECM, has not the attribute of viability' viable or

	nonviable does not relate to the matrix itself. It only relates to the cells. There's no viability in a matrix.
Arthur Coury	I think it hasn't been explored enough, but I defer. So let us put "nonviable" back, and is it that? Okay. And does that look okay to the rest of everybody? Yes, Laura?
Laura Poole-Warren	Just a grammatical thing. I think the "of" before "totally" shouldn't be there. It should be further down. "Implantable prosthesis that consists totally or substantially of nonviable..."
Arthur Coury	Thank you, Laura. Move things around and it happens.
Jiang Chang	Now- sorry. Now you don't need the treated, necessarily, but that's a minor point. David, what do you think?
David Williams	Yes, take it out.
Jiang Chang	Take it out, right?
David Williams	Yes.

(d) Final Definition and Voting for "Bioprosthesis"

Bioprosthesis

Implantable prosthesis that consists totally or substantially of non-viable, human or animal donor tissue

Voting Yes	45
Voting No	2
Abstain	0
Total Votes	47
Number voting Yes or No	47
Percentage Yes Votes	95.7%

The definition achieved Consensus, having more than 75% Yes votes, with absolute number greater than 30.

E Stenosis

(a) Possible Definitions of "Stenosis" Included in Final Program

Narrowing or contraction of a duct or canal

(b) Jiang Chang; Perspectives on "Stenosis" and Suggested Definition

Jiang Chang	Now another term we want to put into discussion is stenosis which defines a narrowing or constriction of a duct or a canal. There are also some other alternatives which says abnormal narrowing of blood vessel or other tubular organ or structure.

(c) Edited Discussion of "Stenosis"

David Williams	I am not sure what abnormal narrowing is because we are looking at, let us say, a stenosis in an artery. We all get it. It is normal when you are getting older. You get stenosis. It is not necessarily abnormal. It is part of ageing. So personally, I don't see the advantage of your second definition compared to the first.
Arthur Coury	And for us it might be pathologic, but we won't get into that. So let us consider the Williams Dictionary term and get rid of the lower term. Do you have a comment? I'm sorry.
John Brash	I guess I would like to ask David why we need to have "constriction" as well as "narrowing" in that definition?
Arthur Coury	Good point.
David Williams	I guess that is there because if you have, let us say it is an artery, you may just have a natural narrowing as opposed to something which is then forming a constriction. I think that's why that was like that.
Arthur Coury	An artery is a muscular vessel and it might spasm and cause a stenosis. Is that what you mean? In part, I believe?
William Wagner	Thrombosis has the pathologic connotation for activation of the hemostatic system and I think stenosis, the way it's used most of the time in the clinical literature, is a pathologic or abnormal narrowing in a blood vessel or other tubular organ or structure. I think it is a good definition and abnormal or pathologic, I think would reflect the state of the literature.
David Williams	I am happy with "pathological."
Arthur Coury	I'm sorry, David. What?
David Williams	I said I'm happy with Bill's comment there including "pathological."
William Wagner	I think it has to be pathological or abnormal or some adjective that conveys that.
Arthur Coury	Let us hide the top definition. Hide it.
Elizabeth Cosgriff-H	Is it necessary to put blood vessel here or keep it more general?
Rena Bizios	I will second that suggestion because, and maybe we can put part of what we had before, an abnormal narrowing or constriction in tubular organs of structures. And we take out the blood vessels as a good example but there always is other tubular organs in the body that may have narrowing or stenosis.
Arthur Coury	I like it and I actually did like the term "constriction" because it could imply a temporary spasm or something like that so I do like that. And take blood vessel out.
Rena Bizios	"An abnormal narrowing or constriction in tubular organs or structures." And that's the end of it.

Arthur Coury	Take the word blood vessel out.
Rena Bizios	It is a tubular organ or tubular structure. Take out the organ. Take tubular structure. If you don't like the organ, I agree with you. Make it tubular structure.
Arthur Coury	And then get rid of the top one.
Joachim Kohn	So Art, I must object to what happened here. Because one person made a comment that another person here made a comment and you just followed that one comment up. We never really discussed or endorsed these changes around, for instance, I've just commercialized a stent and I can assure you that stenosis is largely used in the context of blood vessels. Taking this out significantly confuses the definition. I agree that stenosis can also happen in other ducts, but it has to be part of the definition just as Bill Wagner has said before. And so a lot of editing was suddenly done that was not agreed
Arthur Coury	Before we vote we have to decide on the editing. But Jim.
James Anderson	I have an issue with the word "in." Classic examples of stenosis can occur in the gastrointestinal system secondary to adhesions. And so they form from the outside and not the inside.
Cato Laurencin	I have two objections. The first concerns pathologic. I would say it is a narrowing. Let me just, from experience, I wrote a paper on spinal stenosis. And when I asked for healthy volunteers, they were completely healthy, young, great people and they had CT scans. We looked, and we found that actually the average person had the stenosis ratio, has about 10%, if they're normal, 30-year-old people, no symptoms whatsoever, had about 10% stenosis in L4 and 5. Very bad deal. They were normal and healthy. In other words, over time, that is progressive stenosis and to call it either pathological or abnormal. What happens? Do you do surgery or not? Or do you think it is pathological? Well did you understand that normally, people will have that level of stenosis that is not pathological. It is something that is part of life.
Arthur Coury	This makes sense to me. If everybody agrees, Cato suggests removing both "pathologic" and "abnormal." And really stenosis, yes, Professor Zhang?
Xingdong Zhang	I think this definition is not necessary because this only applies to the natural organ and not biomaterials.
Arthur Coury	But sometimes you use a biomaterial to correct a stenosis and I kind of like the term in there even though it is not a biomaterial based or derived thing although it can be. It can actually be from hyperplasia. From intimal hyperplasia. So I do like keeping the word in there. Other comments? So we'll vote yes or no. Rena?
Rena Bizios	I propose to change the order of appearance of the word "organs" and "structure." Put tubular structure or organ. And that is different.

Yunbing Wang	I think I agree with Professor Zhang's suggestion because for biomaterial related, normally we call it restenosis instead of stenosis. So if we talk about definition, restenosis might be more important for material related issue.
Arthur Coury	I am not a cardiologist. But if a cardiologist notices a 90% constriction in a blood vessel, they might deliver a stent to that.
Yunbing Wang	Correct.
Arthur Coury	And so that is stenosis, that is the narrowing of that blood vessel.
Yunbing Wang	I agree. What I mean is this issue is similar like you talked about heart disease. We gave the definition for heart disease, but we talked more maybe it's a pacemaker related disease. The new issues. So definitely, they need to implant a stent if their stenosis is more than 90%. But for material related issue, the physicians care more about their restenosis. So that definition might be similar to this one, but it is more closely to the medical device made from biomaterial.
Arthur Coury	I do think restenosis is another definition. It is stenosis after something happens.
Yunbing Wang	Do you have restenosis here?
Arthur Coury	I don't think we have that.
Yunbing Wang	My understanding is the best way is, we have stent first and then restenosis. This is more relevant issues.
Arthur Coury	Yes, David?
David Williams	Art, let's be clear so we understand what Yunbing is saying. It is obviously very important in intravascular stents. That by no means is the only place we have stenosis. For example, calcific stenosis in the aortic valve, it is not in an artery but it's hugely important. And my reason for saying let us have this in here … a stenosis is one of the major reasons why we use implanted devices. I agree restenosis we could define as well. But I think when looking at biomaterial terminology, it's good to have some of the most critical pathological or other features there which cause the need for that device. I am not going either way here, but I think we have to be careful not just to concentrate on an artery.
Rena Bizios	We are going to have now definition for stenosis and then for restenosis. Because in my mind, stenosis is something that happens in tissues, as Dr. Zhang brought our attention. Restenosis is something related to the situation after certain implants, for example, vascular implants have been placed. And then they become pathological and abnormal. While in stenosis, pathological and abnormal is not necessarily the main characteristic of what we have in that particular situation.

Arthur Coury	I thought we were going to remove those two terms. This is stenosis. This is not restenosis and I agree with Cato that it is not necessarily pathologic or abnormal. If everybody agrees with that we will remove those two words and get on with the vote. Yes, Bill?
William Wagner	I think there needs to be some notation that it is non-desirable. It is true that you may not intervene for a stenosis because it hasn't progressed to a point, but like thrombosis, it is a non-desirable pathological event and you may allow that pathology to go untreated, but at some point it may cross a threshold where you treat it. So just saying it is a narrowing implies that it could be harmful. These devices are developed to address that when it gets to that point. So I don't know what, maybe pathological is too strong of a word, but something that indicates that it's a non-desirable.
Cato Laurencin	I'm okay with "progressive," but again, if you look at spinal stenosis, 10% of normal people have spinal stenosis in L4 or 5 and I would not call it pathological and I think it is progressive.
Arthur Coury	And to call it progressive, we just don't know that it is going to progress. So I would be …
Cato Laurencin	Stenosis normally is progressive. I mean, I will give you progressive. It is progressive but progressive like something you'll die with instead of for most people.
Rena Bizios	I will leave that to the surgeons and physicians to decide because that is when they have to make that particular decision. But it comes to the point, as Cato mentioned in certain other implications of tubular structures or organs, it is not pathological or abnormal. But if it becomes pathological, if it reaches a case of medical complication that requires intervention, then maybe if we add something like that at the end perhaps we can resolve this particular stalemate.
Arthur Coury	You might reach my age and beyond, Bill, before it becomes a problem even though it is there. So the suggestion of removing abnormal and pathological. Let us try that. If everybody is okay with that, raise your hand. Not everybody. Whoever is okay with that, raise your hand. And who is not okay and would like to have abnormal or pathological remain, raise your hand, please? Okay. The removal is … there were more people for that so we need to vote on this and you vote, right? So let's vote on, let's see.

(d) Final Definition and Voting for "Stenosis"

Stenosis

A narrowing or constriction of a tubular organ or structure

Voting Yes	40
Voting No	7
Abstain	1
Total Votes	48
Number voting Yes or No	47
Percentage Yes Votes	85.1%

The definition achieved Consensus, having more than 75% Yes votes, with absolute number greater than 30.

F Stent

(a) Possible Definitions of "Stent" Included in Final Program

1. A tubular support placed temporarily inside a blood vessel, canal, or duct to aid healing or relieve an obstruction
2. A short narrow metal or plastic tube often in the form of a mesh that is inserted into the lumen of an anatomical vessel (such as an artery or a bile duct), especially to keep a previously blocked passageway open
3. An intravascular stent is a synthetic tubular structure intended for permanent implant in native or graft vasculature. The stent is designed to provide mechanical radial support after deployment; this support is meant to enhance vessel patency over the life of the device. Once the stent reaches the intended location, it is expanded by a balloon or self-expanding mechanisms defined below[1]

(b) Jiang Chang; Perspectives on "Stent" and Suggested Definition

Jiang Chang	The next term is stent. You have two options. One is "a tubular support placed inside a blood vessel, canal, or duct to aid healing or relive obstruction." The second is "a short, narrow metal or plastic tube, often the form of a mesh, that is inserted into the lining of an anatomical vessel, such as an artery or bile duct especially to keep up a previously blocked or narrow passageway open."

(c) Edited Discussion of "Stentz°"

Arthur Coury	You have two definitions up there and I would like to hear a discussion on each of them, on both of them, as you wish.
Maria J. Vicent	I would add also healing or leave or prevent. I would like to include "prevent" as a word.
David Williams	Add healing or prevent?

---

[1] US Food and Drug Administration

Maria J. Vicent	Prevent. Add healing or prevent.
Arthur Coury	Preventing.
Maria J. Vicent	Preventing or relieve an obstruction. It's also preventing, not only healing.
Arthur Coury	You like the top version? Yes?
Nicholas Peppas	It is clear that this term is for the stents that most of us are familiar with. Recently, Professor Bizios and I and a few others listened to some talks about other types of stents that I was not aware of. Vaginal stents. Vaginal stents which are not tubular. And I wonder, David, if you know the word stent is used now in broader sense to support an organ that is falling apart because of elasticity or I don't know what. We can stay with this term, but if we want to be more general, the word tubular may have to be questioned.
David Williams	I am comfortable with that. These are just suggestions. They are not necessarily my definitions. I made these suggestions and I think probably neither would be very good.
Arthur Coury	Nothing more? No other suggestions? And there are, of course, stent grafts which are another form of therapy. But I do believe the stent part of it is valid within the top term.
Joachim Kohn	I would recommend we start with the shorter definition, number one. I think that the number two adds a lot of words whereas the number one is really concise and conveys the message.
David Williams	I would agree with you, Joachim. I much prefer one and if you want to take the word tubular out, I am happy with that too.
Arthur Coury	If everybody likes number one, enough people like number one because we are going to vote on the top definition first. Unless Tim has something to say.
Timmie Topoleski	Well we just spent a long time talking about stenosis, right? And stenosis does not necessarily imply a complete obstruction. So at least in my mind, nothing gets past. So the question is, can a stent be used to relieve stenosis or other narrowing or something like that?
Arthur Coury	So Tim, the term partial obstruction is used an awful lot.
Timmie Topoleski	We could use that.
Arthur Coury	Partial or complete.
Joachim Kohn	Tim made a really important point. I thought it is really nice we have that stenosis part in there so it is a stent to aid healing, prevent, or relieve stenosis. Wouldn't that make perfect sense?
Rena Bizios	The condition by Joachim, we can add an obstruction or stenosis at the end. That is one more word without making very verbose.
Arthur Coury	Yes, it's fine. And I think an obstruction . . .
Rena Bizios	Or stenosis.
Arthur Coury	If you don't say partial, then it is probably implied.

Rena Bizios	Exactly. I like that addition.
Arthur Coury	Does that sound okay to put in "or stenosis"?
Rena Bizios	With the tubular geometric configuration since we have, yes, blood vessels, canals, ducts. They are not necessarily tubular.
Arthur Coury	Does a tube have to be perfectly circular? No, you can have a tube that's all different shapes but it is a hollow structure.
Rena Bizios	Tubular. A support place inside the blood vessel.
Arthur Coury	Do you like that better? I don't like it as much but that is okay enough with people to vote? Taking the word tubular out. I am sorry. We will vote without it first. Okay?
Ji Jian	If you want to use the blood vessel tunnel it must be a tubular support. If you want to involve other stent for other tissues, then you need to include the other tissues. I think, too, now most of the stent I use for the tubular support.
James Anderson	I did not quite catch your example of a partial obstruction? What was it?
Arthur Coury	A partial obstruction is a blockage of part of the cross section of a structure.
James Anderson	If it is obstructed, it's obstructed. If it is not obstructed, it is stenotic. It is pretty simple. So I think that only adds confusion. The second definition, I don't think is necessary - the first definition is fine with the removal of "placed inside a tubular organ to aid healing." Prevent or relieve symptomatic stenosis.
Arthur Coury	Or obstruction.
James Anderson	You do not put these things in without having symptoms
Arthur Coury	Even a total blockage, if you catch it enough, you could run a guide wire through and you could place a stent in. So I would leave the word obstruction in.
William Wagner	I hate to disagree. If they do an angiogram and a patient has symptoms from one artery but not others, they may take the opportunity to go ahead and deal with some other stenoses that may not be symptomatic. For other conditions where they know that there is going to be ongoing blockage in the future from growth of a tumor, they may go ahead and put a stent in prophylactically.
Arthur Coury	I think if we leave it as is, we're okay. Right? What didn't you like?
William Wagner	I objected to "symptomatic." I don't think it adds anything.
Arthur Coury	Just take away the word "symptomatic" and leave it for now.
Arthur Coury	Add obstruction and stenosis. This is a generalized statement. It is broader and it avoids the argument whether it has to be symptomatic or not. It could be potentially symptomatic in the future.

William Wagner	If you have got a major blockage, they will go ahead and treat the major blockage even though you may not be symptomatic.
Timmie Topoleski	Jim, I think we're just defining the device and not why it may go in. Somebody may put it in because it's a malpractice issue, but it is still a stent. I think that's what we want to get to and then argue about whether or not it was properly implanted in a symptomatic patient or a non-symptomatic patient later. Does that make sense?
Jiang Chang	Barring further discussion, let's have a vote on this and then come back if necessary. If we get really close. Let us vote now and catch up.

(d) Final Definition and Voting for "Stent"

Stent

A tubular support placed in a blood vessel, canal or duct to aid healing, or prevent or relieve an obstruction or stenosis

Voting Yes	42
Voting No	0
Abstain	0
Total Votes	42
Number voting Yes or No	42
Percentage Yes Votes	100%

The definition achieved Consensus, having more than 75% Yes votes, with absolute number greater than 30.

G Implant-Related Infection

(a) Possible Definitions of "Implant-Related Infection" Included in Final Program

A host immune response to one or more microbial pathogens on an indwelling implant

(b) Jiang Chang; Perspectives on "Implant-Related Infection" and Suggested Definition

Jiang Chang	Okay, here again we have two similar terms. One's an implant related infection, which is "a host immune response to one or more microbial pathogens on the implant." And the second is "a catheter related infection which is a host immune response to one or more microbial pathogens associated with a catheter diagnosed by both the presence of clinical manifestations of infection and the evidence of colonization of the catheter by microorganisms."

(c) Edited Discussion of "Implant-Related Infection"

Arthur Coury	In the top case you haven't necessarily diagnosed the infection by removing the implant. In the second case it implies that you have.
Carl Simon	The top one does not have to say microbial. It could be any type of pathogen, right? Are there other types besides microbial?
Arthur Coury	Are there any sources of infection that are not microbial?
Jiang Chang	Yes, fungus.
Arthur Coury	Is that not a microbe? Fungus? Is that not a microbe? I thought it was.
James Anderson	I object to the word "host." Is there any other type of immune response?
Arthur Coury	Does anybody object to the removal of the word "host"? Laura.
Laura Poole-Warren	I don't object to the removal of "host," but I am not clear on how the immune response is equivalent to an implant related infection. The implant related infection is basically the formation of a symptomatic biofilm, in essence, on a material or on an implant not the host response or the immune response to the pathogen.
Arthur Coury	I think that is a really good point.
Cato Laurencin	I would just say a pathogen … because fungus are not microbial. Fungus are eukaryotes.
Arthur Coury	Good. I am glad you made me understand that. Call it a pathogen. A microscopic pathogen. I guess all pathogens are microscopic. So, a pathogen. Yes.
Laura Poole-Warren	Can I just check. Earlier on we were talking about an implant not necessarily being indwelling, but partially or completely on the side.
Arthur Coury	In other words, you could have an infection of a topical device. Is that what you mean? Or transcutaneous, percutaneous, topical. This says implant related. David?.
David Williams	Could I just mention here that I put these in the document just as a guide for discussion. I am not necessarily going to defend either of these. I was trying to differentiate between an implant and one of the most important things is the catheter-related infection which is the second part of this. That is why there is the differentiation there. I am not necessarily defending that.
Cato Laurencin	I do have a problem with immune response.
Elizabeth Cosgriff-H	I agree.
Cato Laurencin	I do have a problem with immune response because the response from an implant, in terms of infection, it is a host response that can include immune factors but it is not an immune response. You can have a patient who can be implanted with an implant and have a nickel allergy. If they have a nickel containing implant or

	chromium allergy. That is a true host immune response to that implant versus an infection which is caused by microbes or fungus which creates a different response than an immunological response.
Arthur Coury	What should we say for this?
Elizabeth Cosgriff-H	I would second that. I do not know that the infection is dependent on there being a host response to it. It is more with implant related infection, the purpose or the differentiation is that the implant is acting as a substrate for colonization by one or more pathogens. That is what makes it difficult to treat, the substrate.
Arthur Coury	What makes it difficult to ascertain is if you do not remove that implant to confirm that. Bill?
William Wagner	I think how this would be diagnosed or verified would be a positive culture on a drive line, or from the device, or positive blood cultures that are suspected to be related to the implant. Then at the time of explant that can be verified. It is just what Elizabeth was saying. You have to have the viable microorganisms that you demonstrate are viable by culture on or near the device.
Laura Poole-Warren	Just following up on the host immune response versus infection. The infection relates to the fact that you have an invasion of microorganisms that are actually causing a symptomatic outcome. It's not a colonization. It is actually a symptomatic infection. To say it is a host immune response is actually incorrect. You have a host immune response to the infection, but they are two separate things. I do think we have to make this definition a lot tighter and it might be around invasion of microorganisms related to an indwelling implant. Certainly, that can exacerbate the infection. I do think we have to make that very clear.
Arthur Coury	For sure a colonization is required for an infection, but a symptomatic response is not always required. Is that the idea? If it is not, then this has no relevance.
Rena Bizios	I think we have to specify that these responses are either local or systemic. In my opinion it is very important. The other question. Is the pathogen indwelling on an implant, correct? Or is it correct the way it appears?
Arthur Coury	Those pathogens can be around the implant. They don't necessarily have to be on it.
Rena Bizios	In my opinion it should be indwelling on an implant. If you want to change or remove the word "indwelling" on the implant it's fine. I think we should mention something about the local and systemic type of responses we have to infection. They require medical attention.
Arthur Coury	Does anybody object to the removal of the word "indwelling"? Because an implant is an implant.

Joachim Kohn	I do object a little bit and I would like to suggest a complete reorganization of that sentence because it needs to build from the ground up. I would change it to "an indwelling implant that is colonized by one or more types of pathogens." Start with the implant. I say it again, an indwelling implant that is colonized by one or more types of pathogens.
Arthur Coury	If it is an implant, isn't it indwelling?
Joachim Kohn	Yes.
Arthur Coury	Do you have to use the word "indwelling"?
Joachim Kohn	Okay. I am always in favor of striking things. An implant that is colonized by one or more types of pathogens.
Arthur Coury	That does not imply a pathologic response?
Joachim Kohn	It does not imply a pathological response, but the implant is infected, then it is colonized by bacteria.
Arthur Coury	Right.
Ruggero Bettini	The subject here is of the infection, not the implant. We have to define the infection, not the implant.
Arthur Coury	I totally agree that you can have an infection and it doesn't have to be symptomatic. That infection is either where the cells colonize the implant, or they colonize the vicinity of the implant or both.
Laura Poole-Warren	I am not sure with the definition of infection that you can have an infection without symptoms. I think infection by definition is causing a disease. We could do something like "the process of microorganisms invading the body in association with an implant and causing disease." Something along those lines. That is, in essence, what implant related infection is.
Rena Bizios	What I hear is the possibility of drawing those two definitions in one because they are infected implants.
William Wagner	I like Joachim's simple, clean definition and I would like to strike "the host immune response." Put up Joachim's. Maybe even take a vote on it. Do you want to see if we can?
David Williams	The infection can happen much later. It does not have to happen when the device is placed. It can happen much later. The key definition is viable microorganisms on the device, cultured with the device.
Arthur Coury	And not necessarily causing a pathologic response.
Cato Laurencin	I think I would disagree. It is the response that is there. If you have someone with a chronic catheter they actually get colonized with bacteria. Any person who has a chronic catheter gets colonized with bacteria but because they are colonized for so long they don't have a response. Are they infected? No, we do not call them infected.
Cato Laurencin	You may have an implant in your tooth, one of these metal implants that they are putting in. They are colonized. They are colonized with friendly bacteria, but they are colonized with bacteria. But I do like Joachim's part that says . . . it starts with a

	pathogen that is there, but I also believe it is a response that takes place to a pathogen.
Arthur Coury	There seems to be a consensus that there needs to be a pathologic response in some way or other. We need a few words to add to that statement by Joachim.
Laura Poole-Warren	I guess I would argue that colonization does not equal infection, but having said that, if everybody is happy with that I can live with it. Types of pathogens, whether we would like to actually perhaps use microorganisms instead of pathogens. The most common microorganism that we actually have associated with biomedical device infections is actually considered a non-pathogen, which is staphylococcus epidermidis or coagulates negative staph. Those are commonly found are up everybody's noses, on all of our skin and everywhere.
Arthur Coury	But it can lead to serious consequences.
Laura Poole-Warren	Absolutely, yes.
Arthur Coury	I think we need to say pathologic, pathogens, or something. How do we say causing symptoms or something like that?
Laura Poole-Warren	Cato did you say, causing or resulting in a host response? That would work. If you had an allergic response to the microorganisms, it would appear like an infection.
Rena Bizios	I want to bring your attention something that I learned a long time ago as a junior faculty by the editor Dr. Anderson. There has to be an agreement between the title and the definition. The definition is infection. We are defining infected implant or something like that. We are not talking about infection in this definition. So, something has to change. I like the definition. I do not like the title.
Xiaobing Fu	Our definition is implant-related infection. But all the definitions are immune response. Immune response and infection are quite different. Implanted or not, infection should be defined ... infection caused by implanted materials. It's very simple.
Cato Laurencin	There is an immune portion to the response, but we really do not call it an immune response. We call it an infection response. I know it has immune consequences to it, but we call it a response to the infection rather than the classic type of immune response. We call it an infection response.
William Wagner	There are cases where the immune response is irrelevant. If you have candida infected bioprosthetic valve or VAD, the immune response is not adequate. That is why there is a problem and that embolizes and kills the patient. It wasn't their host response that was relevant. It was the implant centered infection of the candida that grew out of control and caused the problem. So the resulting and host response ... the reason we have a problem is because the host response is inadequate.

Arthur Coury	What can we do here? We are not saying this covers every response, but what can we do?
William Wagner	Why do we have to say it has to result in a host response? It is just the viable microorganisms that are potentially leading to a pathology.
Cato Laurencin	I would answer that to say there is always a host response. Inadequate host response ends in death, by definition. There is a response that takes place whether it is adequate enough to be able to treat it, to stop it or not it is there. It is a way to characterize it because the person will have a fever and chills, etc., which connotes that there is something going on in terms of some sort of host response. Even with the Candida infection, the person will have fever or will present with symptoms of being sick. Those symptoms of being sick are actually the body trying to fight the infection.
Xiaobing Fu	My definition is it is infection caused by implanted materials. There are some response . . . there is no response because we are not causing the immune response. You just defined the infection. Implant is not the infection. Yes. my definition is that the infection is caused by implanted materials. Caused by materials. It is enough. You do not care there is immune response, there is no immune response.
Rena Bizios	I think for the general audience which would benefit from this definition we should include implanted materials which are colonized by one or more types of microorganisms resulting in host responses. I think we need to explain what is happening. The second part of the definition in red can be added, in my opinion. In addition, I think we can put implant related or we can join the catheter and implant. They are both the same. We can throw in the word catheter somewhere in there, so we can have only one definition.
Arthur Coury	I wish we were finishing on a less controversial topic, but this is the end. This is the end of the day for us. We are going to vote on something in just a minute or so.
Rena Bizios	I will just say a couple words with that. I think it is not caused by the implant materials. It is just in that process that happened.
David Williams	Can I just suggest at this point. We've been on this definition for quite some time now. It is not just dinner that is a problem. It is that our attention span is getting a bit difficult here. We are not going to be able to get to "catheter-related infection." That is a hugely important issue in my opinion when we come to look at clinical consequences and responsibilities. What I suggest is that you leave that there. Tomorrow afternoon we come back to both of these fresher. Then we can and then vote on them tomorrow. I think it is a little too late now to do the voting now.

Editor's Note: It was clear that agreement could not be reached on the definition of implant-related infection, nor indeed on catheter-related infection. Time did not permit re-examination of these terms the following day. For the record, the suggested definition for catheter-related infection was as follows:

Catheter-Related Infection

A host response to one or more microbial pathogens associated with a catheter, diagnosed by both the presence of clinical manifestations of infection and the evidence of colonization of the catheter tip by microorganisms

H Other Biomaterial-Based Devices Terms: No Voting, With or Without Discussion

A number of other terms were scheduled for discussion and voting during Session IV but time allowed for only limited discussion and no votes were taken. The definitions proposed by the Plenary Speaker are included here for completeness.

Transcatheter

Performed through the lumen of a catheter

Extracorporeal Circulation

1. Maintenance of blood circulation by means of a device located outside of the body, with blood fed through catheters advanced in an appropriate blood vessel and returning to the body to another blood vessel
2. The circulation of blood outside of the body through a machine that temporarily assumes the heart's functions

Surgical Mesh

A mesh that may be implanted to support tissues or organs

Bridge to Transplant

The concept of using any organ or surrogate device to stabilize a patient before the definitive transplantation of a matched organ

Transplant

Tissue structure, such as a complete or partial organ, that is transferred from a site in a donor to a recipient for the purpose of reconstruction of the recipient site

Graft

Piece of viable tissue or collection of viable cells transferred from a donor site to a recipient site for the purpose of reconstruction of the recipient site

Interventional Device

A device used for diagnosing or treating a condition with the intent of modifying the outcome.

Artificial Organ

A medical device that replaces, in part or in whole, the function of one of the organs of the body

Hybrid Artificial Organ

An artificial organ that is a combination of viable cells and one or more biomaterials

Tissue Adhesive

Any substance that is used to secure wound closure through bonding mechanisms

Device Adhesive

In medical applications, a substance that bonds a medical device to tissue

Surgical tissue sealant

A device that seals tissue against liquid or gas fluid leakage

Bioelectronic implant

Implants that could send an electrical pulse to a major nerve to alter the commands an organ receives, and thereby control its function

Self-powered implantable medical devices

Self-powered techniques based on piezoelectric effect, triboelectric effect, magnetostrictive effect and electromagnetic induction, can convert mechanical energy from ambient environment into electricity. Implantable medical devices (IMDs) including sensors, pacemakers, implantable cardioverter defibrillators, cochlear implant and stimulators for deep brain, nerve and bone, will be self-powered in the future. It means that IMDs can convert biomechanical energy from body movement, muscle contraction/relaxation, cardiac/lung motions, and blood circulation, into electricity for powering IMDs themselves

Untethered soft robotics

Untethered soft robotics are made by special polymer materials, such as dielectric elastomer, hyperelastic membranes and polymer matrix loaded with magnetic microparticles. USR can be driven by electromagnets and electrostatic forces to swim inside and on the surface of liquids, climb liquid menisci, roll and walk on solid surfaces, jump over obstacles, and crawl within narrow tunnels. USRs have potential to be applied in microfactories such as the construction of tissue scaffolds by robotic assembly, in bioengineering such as single-cell manipulation and biosensing, and in healthcare such as targeted drug delivery and minimally invasive surgery

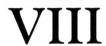

VIII

Biomaterial-based delivery systems

Discussed in Session V

Session V Plenary Presentation: *Nicholas Peppas*
Session V Moderato: *Kazunori Kataoka*
Session V Reporter: *Maria J. Vicent*

A Drug Delivery

(a) Possible Definitions of "Drug Delivery" Included in Final Program

Delivery or release of therapeutic agents

(b) Nicholas Peppas; Perspectives on "Drug Delivery" and Suggested Definition

Nicholas Peppas	We are ready to present to you a very important section, the fifth section in Definitions in Biomaterials, on definitions in drug, gene, contrast agent delivery. And I would like to welcome Professor Kazunori Kataoka, who is going to chair today. I want to also thank Maria Vicent from Valencia, who is the recorder today, and in this particular section we did something different, we worked collaboratively, all together, and there is a fourth person, Professor Ruggero Bettini, who helped.
Nicholas Peppas	I am ready to start with a first term, and I would like to ask Professor Kataoka to stand up and direct. Drug delivery, we propose, "delivery and/or release of therapeutic or diagnostic agents."

(c) Edited Discussion of "Drug Delivery"

Rena Bizios	I think from my perspective it includes all the important aspects, it is very short and to the point.
Laura Poole-Warren	This definition is nice and short however reading it, it could refer to just simply injection of active agents, so basically the delivery of an agent, if you just inject it, so I wonder if we should perhaps

	expand it slightly to incorporate the biomaterial aspect, whether we want to have biomaterial-assisted delivery and/or release of therapeutic or diagnostic agents.
Kazunori Kataoka	You mean put the biomaterials? Biomaterials delivery?
Laura Poole-Warren	Biomaterial-assisted.
Kazunori Kataoka	Biomaterial assistance. Okay.
Hua Ai	I think it is a good definition and just have a small suggestion, because the delivery of drug can be, you know, just the drug, or the diagnostic agent, but they can also be combined. I suggest delivery and/or release of therapeutic and/or diagnostic agents, so put an "and/or."
Nicholas Peppas	The term "and/or" of course we can add it, there's no problem. Laura, thank you very much for your comment. The next slide does include the term "polymer." We felt that the first term needed to be more general because that is really the definition of the whole field and it does not apply just to subcutaneous or to intramuscular or whatever delivery or to the use of polymer or not, but if there is a strong interest in having the word "biomaterials," we can add it.
Kazunori Kataoka	So of course this means not only the injection. Everything. Okay. Any other comments?
Arthur Coury	I wonder if, since therapeutic agents are not necessarily drugs, if pharmacology should be indicated in some way. You could be delivering a therapeutic agent, for example a plate or a screw or something that's even injected that's a device, and that's a therapeutic agent. I mean I think we understand that but how broadly do we want people to understand that it's a drug?
Nicholas Peppas	That's a good comment. Originally, we had the word drug and then all four of us felt that it had to be a little bit broader than a drug because we have peptides, proteins, antibodies and so on, so we felt, actually it was Ruggero's proposal, that we change it to "therapeutic agent," and because we are talking about contrast agents, we added the word "diagnostic agent." If you want to, we can say "of drug, therapeutic and/or diagnostic agents." This could be done too if the committee felt appropriate. Can I see, okay, David.
David Williams	Nick, that was a very helpful comment. I wonder if in a preamble to this session you could identify the difference between drug and therapeutic agent and diagnostic agent, which would be relevant to all definitions and that is a preamble right up front.
Maria J. Vicent	What we consider as a drug usually is a small compound. That is what we understood for all the definitions, and then when we are saying "therapeutic agent," that it was a broader concept, they will include peptides, proteins, antibodies, sRNAs, it is more a concept of bioactive agent or therapeutic agent. Bioactive agent, therapeutic activity. It's a broader concept.

David Williams	Thank you. That could be included in the text somewhere, not as part of a definition, but as to explain these terms, which are relevant throughout. Can we have that as a preamble?
Maria J. Vicent	Yes, will do that.
David Williams	That would be good, thank you.
Nicholas Peppas	Okay, I am adding the word "and/or." Can we have a show of hands how many of you would prefer "drug" before we vote? Is that possible? How many of you would prefer that the word "drug" is added at the beginning? In favor please? Staying with the present term, thank you. Stay with the present term? It is the same. And most of you are abstaining. So, David, what do we do in cases like these?
David Williams	Just as a general principle, as I said yesterday, I prefer not to have the word that's being defined actually in the definition, so I'd rather not put "drug" in there. Keep as you are.
Nicholas Peppas	Okay. Let us vote for that and see. Any other comments?
Kazunori Kataoka	That is a modified definition. "Therapeutic and/or diagnostic agents." Are you satisfied with this?
Nicholas Peppas	Are we ready to vote? Okay, is it open? Is the system open? Please vote for this term.

(d) Final Definition and Voting for "Drug Delivery"

Drug Delivery

Delivery and / or release of therapeutic and / or diagnostic agents

Voting Yes	41
Voting No	3
Abstain	1
Total Votes	45
Number voting Yes or No	44
Percentage Yes Votes	93.1%

The definition achieved Consensus, having more than 75% Yes votes, with absolute number greater than 30.

B Controlled Release

(a) Possible Definitions of "Controlled Release" Included in Final Program

Release of a solute, drug or therapeutic agent from a carrier, system or device in a planned, predictable, and slower-than-normal manner

(b) Nicholas Peppas; Perspectives on "Controlled Release" and Suggested Definition

Nicholas Peppas	Proceeding with the next one. Here we have two possible definitions for, controlled release. First "Release of the solid drug, diagnostic and therapeutic agent from a carrier, system or device in a planned, predictable and slower than normal manner" I know you are not going to like that part. Or, "release of solid drug, diagnostic and therapeutic agent from the carrier, system or device and then depending on the system's properties and characteristics rather than on the compound's mechanical properties."

(c) Edited Discussion of "Controlled Release"

Andrés García	Is the wording "slower than normal" clear to most people? I worry that somebody might say, "What does that mean?"
Nicholas Peppas	Yes, so then maybe we need definitely what is normal. "Normal" is the delivery of the drug without a carrier, so that would be directly by an injection or directly in the stomach but without a carrier present. The implication is the carrier slows down the process, and I must admit, I am presenting it and I'm smiling at the same time because I know there are going to be some questions about what is normal. We could modify it or eliminate that. David.
David Williams	Yes, so I think I mentioned to you, Nick, I did not like "slower than normal." Can't we just delete "slower than normal"? Finished in a planned, predictable manner? I like the first one, if you took that out...
Kazunori Kataoka	Say it again.
David Williams	I like the first definition if you take out "slower than normal."
Maria J. Vicent	Agreed.
Kazunori Kataoka	So just the planned ... and predictable manner. That's fine. Is that what you mean?
Nicholas Peppas	And say a drug, diagnostic therapeutic agent.
Kazunori Kataoka	Any other comments? How about, how do you think of the second? Second one? First one is very simple, second one is maybe more accurate.
Nicholas Peppas	Is there any strong interest in keeping the second one or shall we eliminate it?
David Williams	Just keep the first.
Kazunori Kataoka	Okay.
Arthur Coury	Oh no, I am sorry, this was to the top. Or a therapeutic agent. Is it a drug or a therapeutic agent?
Nicholas Peppas	That is a good comment, and again as Maria pointed out a few minutes ago, drug, we reserve it for small molecules whereas with therapeutic agent we open it up to proteins, peptides, antibodies, whatever else you can imagine. siRNA and so on. If you just voted

| | in the previous one, if you want us to eliminate "drug," we can, although in this particular term the word "drug" does not appear in the … controlled release, it does not say "drug." David, what do you think? |

David Williams   Leave it as it is.

Carl Simon   Another phrase you could possibly add would be "temporally-regulated," because when I think of controlled release I think of time factor in there. "Temporally-regulated." You were saying "slower than normal" so I was thinking of something you could say instead of "slower than normal," you could say "temporally-regulated manner."

Kazunori Kataoka   It does mean in a "planned, predictable and temporally-regulated manner." The proposal is to put "temporally-regulated manner." How do you think, David?

David Williams   I understand what Carl is saying but I do not think that is necessary. I think that explains exactly what we are talking about. And I think "temporally-regulated" suggests you have far more control than you actually have.

Hua Ai   Yes, so also on this comment I agree with David because for some applications there actually is a long-time release, for example, the ring for the birth control and for our applications actually is years long. Maybe just give it that sense.

Nicholas Peppas   I would like to add my comment so that I prefer, Carl, with all due respect, the term "temporally-regulated" opens up a Pandora box. Suddenly temporary, what is temporary, how long and how is it regulated and so on. I don't hear any significant interest in this second term so with your permission I am going to erase the second term. Maria still has the copy so if something happens, we can go back. And here is the term we are discussing.

Arthur Coury   If you add the term "other therapeutic agent," would that address the issue.

Maria J. Vicent   That could be a good point. Because we mentioned drug back to the duplicate.

Nicholas Peppas   The proposal is made that we add the term "other" here.

David Williams   I don't think that is correct grammatically. That is implying the first few are also therapeutic agents but now you are adding another one.

Nicholas Peppas   Thank you. Good comment.

Kazunori Kataoka   Okay. So that is a modified definition. Release of a solute, drug, diagnostic, or therapeutic agent … from a carrier, system or device in a planned, predictable manner. If you are okay, we will move into vote on this. Is it okay?

Nicholas Peppas   Please vote.

(d) Final Definition and Voting for "Controlled Release"

Controlled Release

> **Release of a solute, drug, diagnostic or therapeutic agent from a carrier, system, or device in a planned predictable manner**

Voting Yes	44
Voting No	2
Abstain	0
Total Votes	46
Number voting Yes or No	46
Percentage Yes Votes	95.7%

The definition achieved Consensus, having more than 75% Yes votes, with absolute number greater than 30.

C Pulsatile Delivery

(a) Possible Definitions of "Pulsatile Delivery" Included in Final Program

Solute, drug or therapeutic agent delivery where the release rate is controlled by external triggers, such as magnetic, ultrasonic, thermal, electric, or electromagnetic irradiation, that can produce successive step of increasing and decreasing rates

(b) Nicholas Peppas; Perspectives on "Pulsatile Delivery" and Suggested Definition

Nicholas Peppas	Here is the next definition. What is pulsatile delivery? Solute, drug or therapeutic agent delivery through a formulation that can produce successive steps of high and low rates where the release rate is typically but not exclusively controlled by external triggers, such as magnetic, ultrasonic, thermal, electric or electrical, or electromagnetic irradiation.
Nicholas Peppas	This term is slightly complicated. Suddenly the word "solute" has been added to indicate all kinds of bioactive agents. It can be removed. The word "diagnostic agent" is not there because pulsatile delivery is mostly for drugs and proteins. And I must admit we have added a lot of mechanisms that will lead to this release, which according to the Williams Dictum, probably should not be there, we shouldn't be defining terms based on mechanisms, but it is there to show, at least to remind the participants what are the causes of that, or what are the ways of controlling that delivery.

(c) Edited Discussion of "Pulsatile Delivery"

Rena Bizios	I prefer this statement from the perspective than the one that you had in the book. I leave it to my colleagues who are in the area to decide about the other details, but this is from a presentation or a statement perspective much, much more to the point.
Kazunori Kataoka	Yes.
Carl Simon	Does "pulsatile delivery" include internal physical mechanisms like if you had a layered structure with different solubilities or erosion rates? And so you have one phase and then another phase and another phase being released, does it include that? Because if it does you could say, "Controlled by internal and external triggers" and then add "physical" to your list of mechanisms, if it includes that, but I am not sure if people think that "pulsatile" would include physical mechanisms.
Nicholas Peppas	I see my colleagues in the pharmaceutical field nodding yes. The reality is when we talk about pulsatile delivery, we talked about the result. You are absolutely right. The result can be a layered structure where because of concentration, gradient or solubility difference you have pulsatile delivery. That should be included, and that is an excellent reason why perhaps the mechanisms that are in the last three lines should be eliminated and the word "external" and "internal," how did you phrase it? "Internal and external" could be added.
Carl Simon	Just add "internal or external triggers" and then if you want, you could put physical or something at the end to include dissolution rate.
Kazunori Kataoka	The proposal is "controlled by internal or external triggers." Yes.
Timmie Topoleski	I am a little bit ignorant of this area, Nick. The phrase "through a formulation," is that meant to be a prescribed algorithm where you were talking about a specific frequency and dose?
Nicholas Peppas	You are absolutely right. We use terms used in the pharmaceutical field without having defined them. Formulation is the whole product. The polymer, the additional adjuvants and so on and the therapeutic agent or agents as they are being released, that is a formulation. Your tablet is a formulation, a capsule is a formulation, and I agree with you, it appears for the first time here. Maybe we can "through biomaterial." I don't know my colleagues, I think my three colleagues to my right, Professor Bettini and Vicent and Kataoka are the ones that should make that call. Should we change "formulation" to something else?
Kazunori Kataoka	But it is not too easy to change, right? "formulation" is quite widely used in the field of drug delivery to include all the systems.

Timmie Topoleski	The formulation part is modifying delivery, not the agent. That was my question.
Nicholas Peppas	No, it is not modifying the agent. Your absolutely right. David?
David Williams	Nick, as a brief comment, I do not think you need "not exclusively" — this might be implied by using the word "typically."
Peter Ma	I am just wondering if we can't just eliminate all the different ways. It may be difficult for us to try to predict. There might be more ways to achieve pulsatile release. Rather, we should define what pulsatile delivery is, as long as you achieve that pulsatile or, say, high speed and low speed release, that is a pulsatile delivery, whatever you do. There are more examples, you know, hard to predict everything from there.
Kazunori Kataoka	Okay so how would you like to change the definition?
Peter Ma	That is basically the first part of it. The "typically" and those things after should be removed.
Nicholas Peppas	You are saying something like I am about to show you right now if the system works. Yes, something like this. We have removed all the reasons.
Peter Ma	Even from where, remove all those.
Nicholas Peppas	Oh, remove entirely that.
Kazunori Kataoka	It becomes very simple.
Maria J. Vicent	No, because it doesn't mean the same.
Kazunori Kataoka	But we need some, you know, some way to make this system pulsatile.
Peter Ma	I think the definition is not the way. It's really the results. You have achieved that different rate, fast or slow.
Kazunori Kataoka	The system which can produce successive steps on high and lower rates. That is enough.
Peter Ma	For example, just to go back to the layer by layer, I don't think that is just called a trigger. If we have layer by layer, that is not a trigger. That is just the polymer degrades by its degradation rate rather than by a trigger.
Peter Ma	I feel that triggers are hardly inclusive to every possible way. I would rather remove the prediction of the ways to do it.
Kazunori Kataoka	Your point is just focus on the result.
Peter Ma	Yes. Once you get those results, that is a pulsatile release.
Kazunori Kataoka	So don't put so much about . . .
Peter Ma	The way to do it.
Nicholas Peppas	We have a proposal here, and I am going to change it in a minute. One minute. No, please leave it up.
Nicholas Peppas	Let me decide what we show and what we don't show. One minute please, I am coming back. We have a proposal which

	basically will regain, I am going to change the "solid drug" to "drug, therapeutic or diagnostic agent delivery through "... I will retain the word "formulation" for the time being and if you want, we can define it in a subsequent slide. "That can produce successive steps of high and low rates." I see Professor Bettini, one of my advisors saying yes. Maria, what do you say? You are afraid that by not explaining the causes we are really limiting the definition?
Maria J. Vicent	I think it has a different sense but it is broader.
Nicholas Peppas	It is broader. And if there is another way by which the pulsatile delivery can be pre-prepared, fine, so be it. It is pulsatile delivery. That's how the doctor will see it. What do you think? You think that we are leaning towards that? Thank you, Let me try to summarize.
David Williams	Nick, can I just add one thing there? I understand taking off the specific type of trigger, you don't now need "typically." It's either internal or external.
Nicholas Peppas	Yes. Absolutely. They typically would not be there.
Nicholas Peppas	Let me try to correct now.
Kazunori Kataoka	Any other comments? So the definition become much simple, and based on the results, not for the methodology or procedure.
Nicholas Peppas	So this is the term. This is what we are about to propose as a final version. Please accept it. We need to find a faster way. This is what we are proposing.
Kazunori Kataoka	Okay. So this is a modified definition. It's become much simpler. "Drugs, therapeutic or diagnostic agent delivery, through a formulation that can produce successive steps of high and low rates." Everybody satisfied? Then we are moving to vote.

(d) Final Definition and Voting for "Pulsatile Delivery"

Pulsatile Delivery

Drug, therapeutic or diagnostic agent delivery through a formulation that can produce successive steps of high and low rates

Voting Yes	46
Voting No	2
Abstain	1
Total Votes	49
Number voting Yes or No	48
Percentage Yes Votes	95.8%

The definition achieved Consensus, having more than 75% Yes votes, with absolute number greater than 30.

D Zero-Order Release

(a) Possible Definitions of "Zero-Order Release" Included in Final Program

Constant release of drug over time

(b) Nicholas Peppas; Perspectives on "Zero-Order Release" and Suggested Definition

Nicholas Peppas	The next term is an important term for our field. As you know, for many years, the development of new types of formulations, and drug delivery systems, was done because we could achieve a constant rate of release. Constant rate of release in our field has a very special term, "zero order-release." So zero-order release is "constant release of a therapeutic agent over time," or it could be "release of a therapeutic agent over time at constant rate."
Nicholas Peppas	Our Welsh friend, David, will tell us which one sounds better in English, and Maria has proposed that perhaps we make it broader and call it bioactive agent, meaning all agents. That could include also non-pharmaceutical, non-biomedical agents. Things such as, as they are known in our field, molluscicides, pesticides, anything that affects the environment. Your call.

(c) Edited Discussion of "Zero-Order Release"

David Williams	Nick asked me which is preferable as far as the grammar is concerned. I think the second one is preferable, because the first one says "constant release," rather than a "constant rate of release." So I think the second one is better.
Nicholas Peppas	Okay.
Arthur Coury	Is a contrast agent a therapeutic agent or a diagnostic agent, or should we include diagnostic in that?
Nicholas Peppas	Diagnostic. However, for contrast agent, I am not aware of systems that have a constant release of a diagnostic agent. So, that is why it is excluded.
Kazunori Kataoka	And how does it go, "bioactive agent" instead of "therapeutic agent"?
Peter Ma	There could be other agents that are not really therapeutic. In agriculture, there are things which are not therapeutics, that are released. There are colors, they are released constantly. Flavors, or things like that. It is not really for therapeutic or biological purpose.
Kazunori Kataoka	Absolutely. Actually, there should be some, other than therapeutics, in the agriculture field.
Peter Ma	Right. It could be others.

Nicholas Peppas	Okay. This is what is being proposed recently. For therapeutic agent over time at constant rate, and of course we talked about contrast agent. We did discuss briefly bioactive agent and pesticides and so on.
Kazunori Kataoka	What do you think about pesticides?
Nicholas Peppas	Pesticides. I don't know. Whatever the participants want.
Kazunori Kataoka	So in that case, maybe bioactive agents, is that also include pesticides?
David Williams	Nick, we are not talking about agricultural pesticides.
Nicholas Peppas	That's right.
David Williams	You said at the beginning the terms were biomaterials related- that's implicit in these definitions.
Nicholas Peppas	So why are we suddenly adding something else? You are right. I think we should keep it like this.
Peter Ma	Could choose just "therapeutic or other agent."
John Brash	I would prefer to see the word order changed to read "therapeutic agent at a constant rate over time."
John Brash	It is not just English. It is the sense of the definition. I think the constant rate is what requires to be emphasized. In chemical kinetics, "zero order" means the reactant concentration is raised to the power zero in the rate expression.
Nicholas Peppas	So, John, you want it like this?
John Brash	I want it like that.
Nicholas Peppas	Like this.
Timmie Topoleski	On that same point, do you really need to say "over time," since rate is change of concentration with ... It implies time, right?
Nicholas Peppas	Yes, but that rate is constant, and the question is constant for how long over time? Over time of application.
Timmie Topoleski	Constant means always constant. I am just suggesting you shorten a tiny bit.
Nicholas Peppas	Why are we shortening only in this section? I personally feel comfortable with this.
Kai Zhang	I noticed that you guys picked drugs, and therapeutic agent in some of the definitions and some you just left all the drugs. For example, this one you left all the drugs. So why drug is not in this definition but the others?
Nicholas Peppas	No reason, because it becomes redundant. But anyway, if you want me, I can add it back.
Kai Zhang	I was just thinking from the whole session, consistency. I think David probably addresses it this afternoon, but we need to know a reason. If it is redundant, we just get all together or we just use one term. So if it is therapeutic agent, I understand. Maria explained

	that. When the small molecule for drug and therapeutic agent could be different ones. But I do want consistency.
Nicholas Peppas	It is not a matter of debating. I can add drug. But how do you feel?
David Williams	I understand what you are saying, Kai. But I think here I am quite happy with that because the emphasis is on the zero order rather than on any other mechanism. I do think we should leave "over time" in. I understand again what you are saying, but you took out "over time," that includes having an agent in a syringe which you deliver constantly over two or three seconds. That is not what I think you are talking about.
Nicholas Peppas	So we are talking about leaving it like this, perhaps removing one space before the period. And if there is no more discussion, we are ready to vote.

(d) Final Definition and Voting for "Zero-Order Release"

Zero-Order Release

Release of a therapeutic agent at a constant rate over time

Voting Yes	46
Voting No	2
Abstain	1
Total Votes	49
Number voting Yes or No	48
Percentage Yes Votes	95.8%

The definition achieved Consensus, having more than 75% Yes votes, with absolute number greater than 30.

E Intracellular Delivery

(a) Possible Definitions of "Intracellular Delivery" Included in Final Program

Drug or therapeutic agent delivery of agents to specific compartments or organelles within the cell.

(b) Nicholas Peppas; Perspectives on "Intracellular Delivery" and Suggested Definition

Nicholas Peppas	Now we are going to the next term, which is one that all of you will appreciate. There are many cases where we have a drug or therapeutic agent that actually has to be delivered inside the cell. So we have a term for "intracellular delivery." Delivery of drugs that are critical diagnostic agents within the cell or to specific cell components or organelles.

(c) Edited Discussion of "Intracellular Delivery"

Bikramjit Basu	Can we add "within a target cell" at the end? And also add "delivery of solute and drugs"? Because in other definitions, we have used "solute and drugs."
Nicholas Peppas	The second one, I removed the word "solute" the one time we had it, so we do not have it anywhere. The first one, since Maria and Ruggero were the ones who proposed this specific here, how would you feel about this?
Ruggero Bettini	"Within a target."
Nicholas Peppas	"Target cell."
Peter Ma	I do not have really substantial suggestion, but I thought maybe change "within" to "into."
David Williams	I agree with Peter on that one. If you have "within," it implies you are only delivering the drug into the cell, nowhere else. I think you are talking about a delivery which is targeted such that it crosses cell membrane and has activity in the cell.
Kazunori Kataoka	Do you mean you prefer "into"?
David Williams	I suggest not using "within."
Nicholas Peppas	I understood that. Instead use "into." How about the "specific" being changed to "target"? I feel a little bit less comfortable about that. We are defining it in another narrow way.
Brendan Harley	I agree, Nicholas. I think that may be saying you are going to a specific cell whereas it might not be that specific. There are certainly application where we talk about targeting to a specific subclass of cells. But here you are just talking about getting into a class regardless of whether it is a subclass or not, or any cell it gets into contact with or not. I think that this is more generic, without it.
Arthur Coury	In terms of good English, you can't deliver to specific cell components if you do not get into the cell. So, the term "or" doesn't sound exactly right to me. Maybe "including" or something like that.
Nicholas Peppas	I see what you're saying. You noticed we have changed the word to "into"? How if we say "into the cell compartments or organelles"? To have to say "cell and cell compartments"?
Nicholas Peppas	Remove the word "cell" entirely?
Nicholas Peppas	Remove diagnostic agents into cell compartments. David, "the cell compartments" or just "cell compartments"? Without the word "the."
David Williams	Without "the."
William Wagner	I don't know that I like that last change, because you could just generically deliver it intracellularly, without a targeted compartment or organelle. That would be intracellular delivery. Or you could be more sophisticated and be targeting the mitochondria and some other organelle. Both would be intracellular delivery.

William Wagner	If you consider "intracellularly" as a compartment, but I think it is, the way it was before it captured that more generic kind of intracellular, as well as specific targeting within organelles. Whereas this same way, it seems like it is just targeted to substructures within the cell and specific compartments.
Arthur Coury	And what's I meant, that it is not "or," it is "including" or possibly "including."
Nicholas Peppas	Bill, I can see your point. My point is that when the word is used in a general term, the inventor or the author does not determine a specific compartment, a specific portion of the cell, or anything. So it could be everywhere.
Nicholas Peppas	Art, you are saying "into the cell, including the cell compartments." How do the participants feel about that statement? It sounds a little bit cumbersome to me. "Cell, including the cell compartments."
William Wagner	Would you consider "mitochondrial-targeted drug delivery" to be intracellular delivery?
Kazunori Kataoka	I believe so, yes. It is inside the cells.
Nicholas Peppas	People do that, yes.
William Wagner	And then, or more generic, just at pH whatever, it gets brought into the cell. That is intracellular delivery. I like the way it was before, captured it . . .
Nicholas Peppas	You like it the way it was before.
Nicholas Peppas	Let's go back "into the cell" or "cell compartments" or "including cell compartments"?
Kazunori Kataoka	"Into the cell."
Maria Vicent	Yes, "into the cell."
Nicholas Peppas	Nothing else? I am ready to erase the rest.
Kazunori Kataoka	Just "into the cell"? David? Do you have any comment?
David Williams	It seems to me we have lost all specificity on that now. It can be anything. Any drug delivery, if you have now taken away some of those features. But I think, let me see it again on the screen . . .
Kazunori Kataoka	So that should be some strong intention to deliver into something
William Wagner	I think we need to avoid where we have two words and we just basically redefine those words, like "intracellular delivery," "delivery of things intracellularly." Obviously, it is not quite that simple, but I think there is a tendency, when we simplify out some of these, to just redefine those words.
Nicholas Peppas	David, what Bill says is that now it sounds like we took the term and just reversed it. That's it.
David Williams	Yes, I am reasonably happy with it. I am just wondering where this term will be used now.

Elizabeth Cosgriff-H	I think maybe "cell compartments or organelles," because nucleus is not an organelle, right? Is it? The cell nucleus is a separate compartment, so I would just get rid of "into the cell," and just say "into cell compartments or organelles," because they are all inside the cell.
Nicholas Peppas	David, I think we need to have a term defining what intracellular delivery is.
Elizabeth Cosgriff-H	Or cytosol. You can add cytosol.
Nicholas Peppas	Ah. That will answer David's general point And it better as something a little bit more restrictive.
Ruggero Bettini	May I suggest "delivery of drugs, therapeutic agents through cell membranes." So that includes the external membrane and the other membranes within the organelles.
Kazunori Kataoka	Yes. "Through cell membrane," you mean. But is that also include such processes like endocytosis?
Ruggero Bettini	In this way, we do not have to repeat what is in the title, and it is more specific. So it implies that you have to pass through the cell membrane to deliver something into the cell or into the nuclei or organelles.
Nicholas Peppas	For me, when I deliver siRNA, I deliver it into the cell. I don't just pass the membrane. I can pass membrane, get out some other way without really doing anything to the cell.
Nicholas Peppas	We really need to just focus then. Yes.
Deon Bezuidenhout	To avoid repeating of the word "cell," do "the cell or its compartments or organelles." To avoid the repeat of the word "cell," can we just use "its"? So "into the cell or its compartments or organelles."
Kazunori Kataoka	"Into the cell or its compartments."
Nicholas Peppas	So the proposal is "delivery of drug therapeutic or diagnostic agents into the cell or its compartments or organelles." How does this sound?
Hanry Yu	Organelles are compartments. So, cytosol is a compartment. There are some repeats here. It might be better to say "into the cell compartments." That would be okay.
Kazunori Kataoka	So, you mean direct to cell? Just into the cell compartment?
Hanry Yu	Yes, yes. Just into the cell compartments.
Joachim Kohn	Could you tell me whether there is any drug that you know of that ultimately is not delivered into the cell in some way or another?
Nicholas Peppas	Yes, there are many drugs that will come through the epithelial cells and then it will be metabolized, never get into the cells.
Peter Ma	Some of the drugs could just interact with cell surface like in the receptors. For some others they have to get inside the cells to function.

Joachim Kohn	Isn't it correct that, perhaps I'm mistaken, most of the drugs will ultimately end up in the inside of some cell in their passage through the body?
Nicholas Peppas	Yes, but they may not arrive in the original form. They may be modified, or they may be metabolic compounds.
Joachim Kohn	So, the point I am trying to drive is intracellular delivery, I think, implies the intentional delivery.
Joachim Kohn	Intentional or planned or desired, as compared to what happens to a large number of drugs who just end up in the compartment anyway.
Nicholas Peppas	That's correct.
Joachim Kohn	That was the point I wanted to make.
Kazunori Kataoka	So, that means, for example, you put some planned delivery?
Joachim Kohn	And so basically, intracellular delivery is the intentional delivery of diagnostic agents into the cell or its compartments.
Nicholas Peppas	So you want to put the word "intentional delivery" at the very beginning?
Joachim Kohn	Yes. Intended or intentional as compared to the fact that I saw a large number of drugs some way end up in the interior of cells anyway even if it is not intended because somehow they get metabolized.
Nicholas Peppas	Let me suggest something so that we take a vote, although I think it would be terrible if we don't have a definition on cell delivery.
Nicholas Peppas	Let me suggest "delivery of drugs or diagnostic agents intended for delivery into the cell."
Kazunori Kataoka	Always in this we intend to deliver throughout this carrying. Although some system may release drug outside of the cell and drug itself make entry into the cell. So in that case that is not intracellular delivery, but inter cell delivery means we need some carrier and directly transport the drug into the cell.
Deon Bezuidenhout	The definition is targeted to specific delivery of drugs?
Nicholas Peppas	David you have suggestions? I don't want to lose this term.
David Williams	I agree. I think the Joachim is correct. We have a definition which is fairly specific to the cell type into which we are engaging. Intended or specified, something like that, should be in there. Maybe delivery of drugs, therapeutic or diagnostic agents into specified or target cells and I don't know if we need anything else after cells.
Nicholas Peppas	I would suggest then we try "to specified cells." I am willing to even say "including cell compartments." We don't want that to specified cells.
Nicholas Peppas	So if you have Crohn's disease, you want it to be delivered in those cells. Period.

David Williams	Period. Right. The definition does not need to say which compartment it eventually gets to.
John Brash	To cover Joachim's point I would suggest "delivery of drugs, therapeutic or diagnostic agents directly into the cell or cell compartments."
David Williams	What does directly mean?
John Brash	Right into the cell, the point was no matter the manner you formulate to deliver the drug, the drug will go into the cell, but if you say directly I think that would suggest to me that you are delivering it right to the cell. This is what we want to convey I believe.
David Williams	The word "directly" I think has several different implications. It also seems to me that it doesn't go anywhere else. It doesn't go through any other tissue compartment to get to the cell.
Nicholas Peppas	With all due respect to the colleagues, I think we are making it more difficult than what it's supposed to be. We are talking about delivering to the cells to treat diseases. Joachim, yes everything can go into cells, but not in an active pharmacologically active form. We wanted to go into the cells to treat a disease. If certain fragments in any other application end up getting into the cells, that I would not call intracellular delivery. A company would not sell a product because certain metabolites get inside some of your cells. I like "specific." I think David proposed this. It doesn't define which specific but if you are working with Crohn's Disease you know what specific cells. If you're working with IBDs you know which specific cells, and we leave it at that. I like John your definition, but it says deliver directly. Will it be active?
Nicholas Peppas	Sometimes in this delivery it takes about two, two and a half hours to have the delivery into the cells which is the chronological.
Peter Ma	It also could be first to adhere to the cell membrane and then to internalize. In some way it is not directly sent there, but we can consider it as still intracellular delivery.
Nicholas Peppas	Yes, we receive the final version when I am in the final version. Delivery of drugs, diagnostic agents, how do you say it? David?
David Williams	Into specific or preferably into specified cell. No specific.
Kazunori Kataoka	It was specific. Into the specific cell, period.
Kam Leong	Then you need a linkage. Then you will be targeted cell.
Kam Leong	But if it is just intracellular delivery maybe the delivery, the first line intracellular compartments specifically or non-specifically. That would cover going into the cells anywhere or if you want to target the nucleus, mitochondria, you could also do that but if you want to go into particular cell types.
Kazunori Kataoka	Particular cell type is most of the time. It is cellular targeting but intracellular means or specifies something is in your cell. That is your point. How do you say?

Nicholas Peppas	I think most of the terms we have taken care of the first day have been somewhat general. Within to identify the articular disease or particular treatment, with the exception of minor things like stents and so on. Why are we suddenly putting much higher level of definition for drug delivery? I am willing to agree with everything you said. There will be always a possibility for the drug to go somewhere else, to be broken down. Not to be active. To be less pharmacologically active.
Marie J. Vicent	Could we add at the end to agree with some of the comments in the specific cell to trigger therapeutic output.
Kazunori Kataoka	Trigger a therapeutic?
Marie J. Vicent	Or achieve a therapeutic effect. But as you say for sample it is not the same intracellular delivery. We want to deliver drugs that are pharmacologically active.
Kai Zhang	The current version looks good to me.
Nicholas Peppas	I would recommend we try to vote for this.
Kazunori Kataoka	Yes. So this become very simple definition. I think it simply is very important. So wrap up and move into both.

(d) Final Definition and Voting for "Intracellular Delivery"

Intracellular Delivery

Delivery of drugs, therapeutic or diagnostic agents into specific cells

Voting Yes	30
Voting No	15
Abstain	0
Total Votes	45
Number voting Yes or No	45
Percentage Yes Votes	66.7%

The definition achieved Provisional Consensus, having more than 50% Yes votes.

F Therapeutic Agent

(a) Possible Definitions of "Therapeutic Agent" Included in Final Program

A substance used to treat a disease or other medical condition

(b) Nicholas Peppas; Perspectives on "Therapeutic Agent" and Suggested Definition

Nicholas Peppas	Let us go to this one. Let us hope this will pass easily. Therapeutic agent. A substance used to treat a disease or other medical condition.

(c) Edited Discussion of "Therapeutic Agent"

Rena Bizios	In view of the comment made at the very beginning of this session, and the characterization or definition of what is an agent and what is a drug, I think this particular definition has to be little bit more carefully reviewed and revised. We have to make that clear because I heard a very clear distinction by the colleagues in the field of what a drug or a therapeutic agent is. I do not see it in this definition.
Nicholas Peppas	Do you have Rena a possible different term? A compound-
Rena Bizios	I'm sorry I do not.
Nicholas Peppas	Small or large molecule?
Rena Bizios	I defer to the colleagues in the field because they know the terminology. I don't know the terminology in the field, but it was something that impressed me that there was a clear distinction between "drug," that's what we made at the very beginning of this session, and "therapeutic agent."
Nicholas Peppas	The reason "therapeutic agent" is defined like this here, and all four of us talked about it extensively, is because we wanted to cover the therapeutic action of the compound. Whether the compound is a very small molecular weight molecule or a large molecular weight molecule or a protein or antibody and so on it is active because it creates conditions for therapy of a particular disease and that was the whole idea. So we used the word substance which was used in the pharmaceutical field. It was proposed by one of us four and the other three did not revise it. It is a word used in the pharmaceutical engineering and science field very openly. I agree with you it does not define small or large molecular weight or types of molecules but here the idea is to define the therapy. The therapeutic characteristic of the compound. That is all it is.
Arthur Coury	So did we all appreciate that that could include a device, per example hyaluronic acid injected into the knee for osteoarthritis is considered a device but I think it would fall under this definition very well, and I don't object to the breath of this, but I hope we all appreciate that.
Nicholas Peppas	I must admit we did not presume that.
David Williams	I am not sure we are in position to be defining this by itself as one of our terms. Right from the beginning I said I think there should be a preamble stating what the conventional view of drug, of therapeutic agent, without us voting on this as that is what the literature says. I would rather not have this as one of the terms we are defining. As long as we have that preamble which I mentioned.
Nicholas Peppas	We could have that preamble. Is this something that others-

Kai Zhang	Yes I have the similar feeling about what Art just commented. I am looking at this I don't know are we looking at a drug, are we looking at a medical device or we just don't care because I couldn't tell just by this definition.
Nicholas Peppas	Okay. I guess we are willing to withdraw this one and discuss it further if that's what you want. Any strong feelings to continue discussion?
Kazunori Kataoka	Okay maybe move to vote.

(d) Final Definition and Voting for "Therapeutic Agent"

Therapeutic Agent

A substance used to treat a disease or other medical condition

Voting Yes	41
Voting No	1
Abstain	0
Total Votes	42
Number voting Yes or No	42
Percentage Yes Votes	97.6%

The definition achieved Consensus, having more than 75% Yes votes, with absolute number greater than 30.

G Programmable Delivery, Sustained Delivery, Immediate Delivery

(a) Possible Definitions of "Programmable Delivery, Sustained Delivery and Immediate Delivery" Included in Final Program

Programmable delivery
Controlled release of solute, drug or therapeutic agent at desired time points
Sustained delivery
Release of a solute, drug or therapeutic agent at slow rate over a long period of time.
Immediate delivery
Release of solute, drug or therapeutic agent instantly upon administration

(b) Nicholas Peppas; Perspectives on "Programmable Delivery, Sustained Delivery and Immediate Delivery" and Suggested Definitions

| Nicholas Peppas | I am about to present three terms together, explaining to you that the field of drug delivery is a very litigious field and, in that field, we have many patents. And the patents define things in different ways. We may decide to define those terms today. Probably it is |

	not going to affect the scientific field. If you can believe it, it can affect lawyers. It will affect the legal field.
Nicholas Peppas	So here are the terms. They appear in many patents. "Programmable delivery," "sustained delivery," "immediate delivery." We would like to hear your comments. If you think this is something that should be discussed or just eliminated. And we go further on the scientific terms.
Nicholas Peppas	As you can imagine, the biomaterial plays a role here. Of course, you know, in immediate delivery the biomaterial, obviously is going to disappear very fast. In a sustained delivery, it's going to be present for longer time. But how do you feel? How do the participants feel?

(c) Edited Discussion of "Programmable Delivery, Sustained Delivery and Immediate Delivery"

Rena Bizios	The term "slow delivery rate," in my mind, does not jive with sustained delivery, of how we understand sustained anything these days. Is there another word that can substitute the "slow rate"? The slow, the term, the adjective "slow." Sustained delivery does not necessarily mean slow.
Nicholas Peppas	That is a very good point, because you are thinking of sustained ability as we use it right now in the field. Sustained as it appears in patents means over a longer period of time. It defines the chronological characteristic, the time characteristic of the release. It does not define sustainability again.
Rena Bizios	In this particular context though, we can say that at a predictable, desirable, something rate over a period of time, because that is what it could be, slow, could be intermediate rate, could be high rate as long as it is maintained over a long period of time. Am I correct in reading it that way.
Peter Ma	For the first one, I thought we say at desired time points. We should kind of give you the indication that it happens at discrete times, not in a continuous way. But I think that we should include continuous ways. So the programmable is more like predetermined, I think. That's predetermined delivery, or in a predetermined fashion.
Kazunori Kataoka	You prefer "predetermined delivery"?
Peter Ma	Right. Predetermined.
Kazunori Kataoka	So that is a definition of delivery.
Peter Ma	But it could be continuous, not just desired time points. This could be continuous.
Arthur Coury	If you would use the word for sustained delivery at a specified rate over a planned period of time, I wonder if that is still

	predetermined, you can always determine it exactly, but you could plan a period of time and you could specify the rate of delivery.
Arthur Coury	Yes. Slow rate. How would you define slow? How would you define long? But if you specify the rate, and you plan the period of time, at least you are planning for it and if you can't prove it is going to go that long.
Kai Zhang	Nick, I thank you and your group for picking all those words, the terms. I think this is what the definition meeting is about. The confusing ones and the debatable ones. I think in the legal documents and for the legal cases, we as a group, as a union. We should have a voice; they should hear our voice. So I think this is the meaning of the definition, because it is very important. I am not an expert of delivery, but I hope we have a very good definition on those terms and let people hear our voice.
Ruggero Bettini	I understand Rena's point concerning the slow rate. But consider that this is somehow implicit, because if you have a certain dose and you only increase the time over which you release the dose, you have obviously to slow down the rate. Otherwise it would not be possible to have the same rate for a prolonged period of time. So maybe we can remove the term "slow rate" and keep it as an implicit point.
Serena Best	I was just going to suggest the word either "intended" or "defined."
Joachim Kohn	I would like to endorse this. From a legal perspective, slow rate and long-term are all undefined and relative terms. So the definition does not really help in any way. It is a nice definition from a science perspective. "Slow" and "long" are simply legally useless.
Joachim Kohn	And so what I think is that we either stay, Nicholas, that we either stay silent on this or we really try to avoid terms that are, that at the end don't help. And I think some of us have done enough legal work to understand how the lawyers will have a feast on this.
John Brash	I was going to suggest that the word "slow" should be replaced by "constant." But I guess based on the comment that we heard from Ruggero, which then suggests that you might want to change the rate at some point during the delivery process, "constant" would not apply.
Cato Laurencin	So my view is in terms of sustained delivery versus controlled delivery. And maybe this is just an old-school view. Controlled delivery is delivery that is determined by a vehicle that influences either the drug or the solute.
Cato Laurencin	Sustained delivery is delivery that is determined by the drug itself, either complexation of the drug with a salt, interactions with an excipient that changes the drug. So, if you look at, in the

pharmaceutical industry, all the drugs that have SR after them, it is because they have actually taken the same drug that they have, it's going off patent, and they did a complexation with a salt and make it a sustained release formulation that takes place over time. Or they add a different excipient system that they placed in the drug in terms of its packaging that now allows it to release at a slower rate.

Cato Laurencin	So sustained delivery, you know, change in the drug, complexation, normally with salts or bases. Controlled delivery, the vehicle is actually determining the release.
Nicholas Peppas	Thank you very much. I would like to make a few comments based on some of the things that are said.
Nicholas Peppas	The delivery can be slow or fast, depending on the application. I don't know how you are familiar you are but in the last two years, there has been a tremendous exploration in the area of sublingual drug delivery to help patients who have cancer and where you want to give them fentanyl or other compounds immediately. Immediately means in 10 seconds. Suddenly the delivery time is 10 seconds. What do you define as slow and fast? The important thing is you want to give it to the patient immediately.
Nicholas Peppas	In other cases, you may want to give in two minutes, three minutes. In an ocular application, in the eye, if you can deliver it for half an hour, that is a slow release device. So what I am saying is that we are trying to cover here a large number of terms. Not only implants. Not only transdermal systems, but also other systems.
Nicholas Peppas	Related to Cato's statement, I wanted to say I wish it were true, Cato, but if you have seen patents, people use the word "sustained" with an excipient, with a polymer, with a biomaterial in it. A less designed biomaterial, maybe a hydroxy-propyl-methyl cellulose, an HPMC. But they use it with that.
Nicholas Peppas	This is only to clarify a little bit, but I want to go back to what Joachim said. If you feel that suddenly this is becoming too complex, let us drop it. We have some other terms that are important to define today.
Elizabeth Cosgriff-H	Maybe just putting it in the context of the clinical outcome, at a predetermined rate relevant to the clinical efficacy or outcome, and then it is dependent on what you're trying to do - what the application is, defines what slow is. So if you say predetermined, I think, as Peter had suggested, and then make it relative to the outcome.
Rena Bizios	This is a good suggestion by Elizabeth. It will extend the definition a little bit and make it a little bit longer, but it will go to only one word substituting "slow." I will go with this suggestion, which I

	think was made by Serena. Instead of "slow," use "defined," because then, in my mind, it refers to what you, Nicholas, just said about that requirement. So, delivery in the cases of various patients.
David Williams	Nick, as you know, I do a lot of litigation work as well. I am entirely in agreement with Joachim here. If we have the definitions that are here, which are not helpful in court, in other words, they are too imprecise, then we are doing a great disservice. My suggestion is to avoid all three of these in our document.
Ruggero Bettini	In my view programmable and sustained delivery are specification of controlled release. They are included in the general term of controlled delivery.
Nicholas Peppas	Can we put aside this particular slide and not discuss it any further and not vote?
Nicholas Peppas	Okay. That's how we will do.
Kazunori Kataoka	Okay. Not vote.
Nicholas Peppas	We will not vote it and I will eliminate it.

Editor's Note: The discussion was terminated at this point and no final definitions were proposed and no votes taken. This matter is discussed again in the final Chapter of these Proceedings.

H Other Biomaterial-Based Delivery Terms: No Voting, With or Without Discussion

A number of other terms were scheduled for discussion and voting during Session V but time allowed for only limited discussion and no votes were taken. The definitions proposed by the Plenary Speaker are included here for completeness.

Bioadhesive polymer or carrier

A polymer, synthetic or natural, that can interact with or bind to tissue

Mucoadhesive polymer or carrier

A polymer, synthetic or natural, that can bind to the mucus or the mucosa

Targeting

A process of drug or therapeutic agent delivery only to the desired site of action

Gene therapy

The transplantation of normal genes into cells in place of missing or defective ones for the treatment of genetic disorders

Gene delivery

Delivery and introduction of foreign genetic material (i.e., DNA, RNA) into host cells

Chemotherapy

Treatment of cancer by drugs that destroy cancerous cells/tissues

Drug Eluting (device)

A device which (slowly) releases a drug to prevent cell proliferation

Immunotherapy

A treatment which elicits or suppresses an immune response

Liposomes

Spherical vesicles composed of one or more phospholipid bilayers

Microneedle

A micron-scaled device used to penetrate tissues

Micelles

Aggregates of self-assembled amphiphilic molecules

Nanoparticles

Particles at the sub-micron scale

Nanotechnology

The science of manipulating materials at the sub-micron level

Non-viral gene vector

Synthetic or natural vehicles that facilitate gene transfer to targeted cells without degradation of the delivered gene

IX

Biomaterial-based biotechnology

Discussed in Session VI

Session V Plenary Presentation: *Kristi Anseth*
Session V Moderato: *Kam Leong*
Session V Reporter: *Jiandong Ding*

A Biochip

(a) Possible Definitions of "Biochip" Included in Final Program

1. A miniaturized laboratory capable of screening large numbers of biological analytes for diagnosis and detection
2. An array of miniaturized chemical or biological test sites arranged on a substrate so that many tests can be performed simultaneously and with high throughput and speed
3. A hypothetical computer logic circuit or storage device in which the physical or chemical properties of large biological molecules are used to process information

(b) Kristi Anseth; Perspectives on "Biochip" and Suggested Definition

Kristi Anseth	So this is our challenge. We are hoping that we can come up with some definitions that will have consensus for our group. And I tried to cluster some of these concepts that you will see in the pre-reading material. The first area that we wanted to talk about was some of the emerging areas of making miniaturized devices that are very useful in vitro for making measurements. And some of them are called biochips for different types of assays, or microfluidics. Or even more complex systems that combine either devices are microfluidics with growing tissues and integrating biomaterials to make organs or various tissues on a chip. And then we maybe have a foul here in that we added one term that is not in the book that we wanted to talk about. And that is the microphysiological systems.

Kristi Anseth	So for today's discussion, I am just going to present the highlighted "biochips," "organs on a chip," and "microphysiological system." And if time allows, we'll come back to these three because these I think they have been more well-defined in current literature. So if there's an objection and somebody wants us to discuss one of these three, I am going to hold off and if time allows, come back to it.
Kristi Anseth	All right so the first one with the "biochip." We have three different alternatives. But they all relate to making a miniaturized device for diagnostic and detection of different types of analytes. So the first, "a miniaturized laboratory capable of screening large numbers of biological analytes for diagnosis and detection." The second is "an array of miniaturized chemical or biological test sites arranged on a substrate so that many tests can be performed simultaneously in high throughput and speed." So this one emphasizes more the processing; this one recognizes more what the outcome is. And then the last one, which I'm not recommending, is one that is out there. And it's more about integrating and using biologics and molecules to perform computational functions. So it is not an assay itself. It is part of the device, and is for logical read outs.

(c) Edited Discussion of "Biochip"

Nicholas Peppas	Kristi, I like the first one very much. The only thing I would suggest is the word "laboratory." Different people think differently about this. Can we replace it by "system"? A "miniaturized system."
Kam Leong	Right.
Kristi Anseth	Okay.
Kam Leong	That would be great. Thank you. Can we show a hand on either one or two, and we can focus the energy to find the definition?
Madoka Takai	I think number one is the best for the explaining the biochip. Including the microarray and also the biological computing. So it is biochip including the number two and the number three concept. So I think number one is better to miniaturized testing device.
Andrés García	I also like number one with the suggestion that Nicholas made. I do not like "laboratory," but I think system or something like that would be good.
Brendan Harley	I do not mind one. I like one aspect of number two in that number one focuses on biological analytes whereas number two talks more about what could be a series of chemical or biological tests. I think that some biochip applications might have more than one. So I think if there is a way we can work part of that wording into number one.

Kam Leong	That is a good point.
Brendan Harley	I like the element of number one.
Maria Vicent	Yes, I was going to say more of the same. And also, I like number one. Maybe a miniaturized array system or rationally designed system. And then biological and chemical.
Helen Lu	I was going to say the same.
Hua Ai	I like number one too. But I like the word "high throughput" in number two if it can be integrated in the number one.
Kam Leong	So we will incorporate important terms of two into one and then we focus our energy to refine that.
Bikramjit Basu	Yes, so if the number one definition ends with "for diagnoses and detection with high throughput and specificity "maybe.
Kam Leong	Okay. You can … Can you say that again.
Bikramjit Basu	"For diagnoses and detection for high throughput diagnoses and detection." Yes that is fine.
Kristi Anseth	For "high throughput." Okay so put it here for "high throughput."
Carl Simon	Thank you. I would also add a key feature is a systematic or methodical approach. So maybe you could put "methodically" or "systematically screening." For me, when I have done these types of experiments, my main goal is to try to make things more methodical.
Hanry Yu	Yes, in fact most of the biochips are not "high throughput." The throughput, low throughput, medium throughput is okay. So it should not have the "high throughput."
Carl Simon	I agree with that. They are often not high throughput.
Carl Simon	But they are systematic.
Rena Bizios	For some reason, I don't care for the words "capable" or "able" for inanimate objects. I would suggest a miniaturized system for … Exactly. Thank you.
Arthur Coury	Thank you. I am revealing my ignorance here but do cells get involved in this and where do they come in? Do they not have to be part of the chip or something?
Kristi Anseth	They don't have to be.
Arthur Coury	Okay, but how do the analytes come about?
Kristi Anseth	There are many ways of introducing the analytes. Either the solutions going across the chip or it can be integrated into a microfluidic device.
Laura Poole-Warren	Just on the definition. Since we've removed "high throughput," I think we should probably remove large numbers as well.
Kam Leong	Okay. Screening biological …
Helen Lu	Maybe instead of large numbers, you say multiple biological and chemical test sites?

Kam Leong	Okay. You took numbers off, right? Do you need "numbers" off? Yes. Is "test sites" the right term? The best term? It is. Okay. Good? Can you delete two and three? One more.
Wei Sun	I suggest in the first one to delete the methodical. You know it is a device system for screening.
Carl Simon	Well I think that these systems are usually methodical because you get lots of measurements on the same plate in a side-by-side fashion which to me, is the attractive nature of these systems. They also often get large numbers or multiple numbers. So I think methodical or systematic for me is the number one reason for doing these types of experiments.
Nicholas Peppas	I too agree that the "methodically" has to stay there. It shows a certain sequence and a certain reproducibility also and concern to do it really many times.
Helen Lu	I also like the word simultaneously in definition two. I think because they are screened all at the same time. So I don't know where we would … Simultaneously screened? Yes.
Kristi Anseth	Okay?
Jiandong Ding	So I think that biochip firstly should have some function like a chip. So array, this is a key word. For the array. It is better to be included.
Brendan Harley	For the array, I mean it could have array in there but it is like the high throughput aspect as well is that you could have a high throughput biochip or array-based biochip that we could add an adjective at the front to specify, because I don't think it always has to be an array-based system. It often is but I don't think we necessarily have to say it must be.
Kristi Anseth	Array system or not?
Hanry Yu	Yes. It does not have to be screening, for the purpose of screening. It can be used for testing because fluidic flow and chips and certain things like that are environmentally precise. Not every application involves screening. It might use the term "testing" or "probing" or something like that instead of "screening."
Kam Leong	Testing. Measuring is better.
Hanry Yu	Biological and chemical attributes or properties or something like that instead of test site.
Kam Leong	Okay. Ready? No objection. Let us vote.

(d) Final Definition and Voting for "Biochip"

Biochip

A miniaturized array or system for methodically and simultaneously measuring multiple biological or chemical properties for systematic diagnosis and detection

Voting Yes   46
Voting No   0
Abstain   0
Total Votes   46
Number voting Yes or No 46
Percentage Yes Votes   100%

The definition achieved Consensus, having more than 75% Yes votes, with absolute number greater than 30.

B Organ-on-a-chip

(a) Possible Definitions of "Organ-on-a-chip" Included in Final Program

1. 3D cell-culture models integrated into microfluidic devices to mimic the biological activity, dynamic mechanical properties and biochemical functionalities of a whole living organ
2. A multi-channel, microfluidic device that contains cultured human cells within a controlled microenvironment to recapitulate the molecular, structural, and physical characteristics of a given organ system

(b) Kristi Anseth; Perspectives on "Organ-on-a-chip" and Suggested Definition

Kristi Anseth   The second is about this emerging area of "organ-on-a-chip." The concept is having three-dimensional cell culture models that are usually integrated into microfluidic devices. The first definition emphasizes that but it is "to mimic the biological activity, dynamic mechanical properties and biochemical functionalities of a whole living organ." The second focuses more on the device and it is "a multi-channel microfluidic device that contains cultured cells within a controlled microenvironment to recapitulate the molecular structure and physical characteristics of a given organ." The second is a little bit more device centric and is more about again the outcome. I am wondering if maybe we could just get a quick sense. Does anyone prefer one over two? I kind of preferred one in this sense. One?

(c) Edited Discussion of "Organ-on-a-chip"

Andrés García   I think one is a good starting point. Just to comment, I do not think all of these are necessarily 3-D. I would get rid of the 3-D. And there are some organs/tissue on a chip. I wonder whether we should keep whole living organ. You could say tissues or organ functions or something.

Kristi Anseth	I like how you have it in the bottom one. About giving characteristics of the organ system.
Andrés García	Organ or tissue system, yes I am fine with that.
Hua Ai	For the organ-on-a-chip, should we only include the mimic of normal tissues. The organs, do we include the disease model in this kind of organ chip?
Kam Leong	I would think so.
Kristi Anseth	Yes, so I can modify this; my intent was that you are just trying to mimic. It does not define normal does it, or I think you could mimic a diseased tissue. Or should I include native or diseased?
Andrés García	I don't think you need it but that is where you need "tissue" because if you're trying to look, for example, at a tumor on a chip, that really is not an organ, it is more of a tissue. But I think the way you have it stated could apply to both a normal condition and a pathological state.
Kam Leong	My question is why "mechanical" - does it need to be there?
Rena Bizios	If you don't like the "mechanical," you can go back to the biophysical. And then it is not properties, it is a number of factors of the physical milieu environment or something along those lines.
Carl Simon	I was going to say the same thing. Because when I think of these things, a key aspect is the diffusion issue. So, having physical in there I think is key.
Kristi Anseth	I might suggest "and/or." Because not all of them recapitulate. I think with the environment and/or biochemical functionality, iti s just to indicate it could be some combination.
Kam Leong	Right. So I think we are, we are ready to vote on one. Right.
Kristi Anseth	Thank you.

(d) Final Definition and Voting for "Organ-on-a-chip"

Organ-on-a-chip

Cell-culture models integrated into microfluidic devices to mimic the biological activity, dynamic biophysical environment, and/or biochemical functionalities of a given tissue or organ system

Voting Yes	46
Voting No	0
Abstain	0
Total Votes	46
Number voting Yes or No	46
Percentage Yes Votes	100%

The definition achieved Consensus, having more than 75% Yes votes, with absolute number greater than 30.

C Microphysiological System

(a) Possible Definitions of "Microphysiological System" Included in Final Program
No definition was proposed before the Conference

(b) Kristi Anseth; Perspectives on "Microphysiological System" and Suggested Definition

Kristi Anseth	The third term here is one that may take a little bit of discussion. During the conference, there were some discussions about adding the term of "microphysiological system." This is an area in the US where there are large calls for proposals and research in the area physiological systems. The idea builds on the organ-on-a-chip or a tissue-on-a-chip, but it is really about integrating them. So it is all about interconnections of organs or tissues on a chip, typically using human cells to support physiological evaluations of complex interacting biological systems. That is a little bit clunky. But the intent is that they really provide an advanced in vitro platform that integrates organs on a chip for things like drug screening, disease modeling, and precision medicine, where you can get the interactions between multiple physiological processes. So this is one put forth by Kam so he should get the credit for this definition.

(c) Edited Discussion of "Microphysiological System"

Rena Bizios	I like the second one from my perspective. The only thing I am not quite sure is that precision medicine. Any suggestions for either modification of that "precision" word or another term?
Kam Leong	The old term was "personalized" but the modern term is "precision."
Rena Bizios	Personalized, much better.
William Wagner	I like the first one better. And regarding the second one, I don't know what "advanced" means. It is kind of a cliché term.
Kam Leong	It just means it will take you six to 12 months to make that system.
Brendan Harley	I like the less modified second one. The key thing is integrating the organ-on-a-chip. But I actually like the second half of the first one. You're really looking at the interactions between the complex interacting biological systems as the goal of doing microphysiological models. I like that sort of end of the first one and set up of the second one.
Kristi Anseth	Could I make a proposal? Maybe for this one. So in a dictionary sometimes we have multiple definitions and maybe this one is new enough that there is sufficient synergy to consider having both.
Kam Leong	So you are really going to consider two, we must include two features that this is to be human cell-based. That is the whole point

	of this term. The other is that there is a physiologically relevant flow in the system. Those are the two key features of this term.
Nicolas Peppas	Kristi, throughout the day yesterday and this morning the definitions were, I want to say on simpler things if you know what I mean by that. When we got into more complex things we kind of said, we covered enough. Suddenly I see a term here, I am trying to recognize which devices, which systems are presently in the market or are going to be in the market soon. Who are the investigators working in those systems? Are we suddenly becoming too detailed about certain things that only two or three people are trying.
Kristi Anseth	Well maybe we could take a sense of how many people want to keep discussing this term and potentially coming up with a definition versus how many think it is premature. So how many think we should keep discussing this?
Wei Sun	I think we have the right title for this session - emerging. You know emerging means it is indicated that it is the new future. And there is going to be much happening, my personal view to know this is really booming field. We should keep it in the session.
David Williams	That is why this session is here. Emerging, in the future. When we started off we talked about basically historical aspects of biomaterials and we felt it was very important to look to the future and that is why this session is here. I am very happy to see us move in this direction. I think it is very important. I am always surprised just how many people are working in these areas.
Hanry Yu	Actually with these types of systems there are quite a lot of people working on it. Companies are developing multiorgans on chips and these institutes in Boston have been doing lots this kind of thing. So we have, what I would suggest for this too is we either keep it as it is or as two items. Like yesterday we have multiple entries, definitions. Another possibility, this two can be combined into one as well if you want.
Elizabeth Cosgriff-H	I think just to clarify for me. Maybe interconnections of multiple organs on chip systems using human cells just to differentiate this is multiple organs connected together. I think I lose that when it is "organs on a chip."
Kam Leong	Multiple, yes. Multiple organ system.
Rena Bizios	For my perspective I don't see the need for two definitions. Because there is a lot of overlap. I go with the suggestion that was made earlier of perhaps bringing together these two definitions. One editorial type comment regarding the first definition. We are not doing physiology. We are doing physiologically relevant or pertinent evaluations. With the system if they are relevant and pertinent. Physiologically relevant evaluations.

Hua Ai	So a small question. I saw you have an organ-on-a-chip, organs-on-a-chip. And also organs-on-chips. We just want to make sure which one is most really used in this field.
Kam Leong	Right, that has been suggested by Elizabeth, who simplified it into multiple organ systems. So "multiple organs" would work. They are on the chip. They are in a separate chamber. So you would have a liver chamber, cardiac chamber, connected by flow.
Rena Bizios	Another editorial type question. Is the interconnections or is it interconnected multiple organs?
Kam Leong	Good point. Helen please.
Helen Lu	Pick up multiple?
Helen Lu	I would just add tissues, interconnected tissues or organs on a chip. And get rid of systems.
Kam Leong	Yes, good point.
Bikramjit Basu	So instead of "precision" can we add "personalized"?
Kam Leong	"Precision" I thought is kind of the modern term.
Ling Qin	It's arguable about precision medicine. Precision diagnosis may be, but medicine? If current medicine is not precise, so it's really arguable terms nowadays.
Kam Leong	That's open to debate.
Brendan Harley	For lack of another, do we absolutely need the last part? Drug screening and disease modeling or we could even get rid of all of that. So you're curious about questions relating to the interaction of multiple biological systems.
Kam Leong	I thought you were making the point that this term was so new that it would have to be more explicit to describe what it does.
Brendan Harley	It could be, but once they were curious about if it is precision or personalized, and that aspect could fall under drug screening and disease modeling.
Kam Leong	For drug screening and disease modeling, I think that might work. To cut out the last.
Rena Bizios	This is a new area, perhaps we need that enumeration of certain examples. Because they cover a broad perspective of applications. But whether it is drug-related or precision diagnosis and personalized medicine, all of these things are such a wide spectrum of possible applications.
Kam Leong	But I think Brendan's point is that precision medicine is actually in the category of drug screening.
Rena Bizios	Yes, I heard another definition of precision diagnosis and personalized medicine. Again from an outside, that splitting it into two it will be a little bit more attractive. But if it is a definition which the people in the field use it.
Kam Leong	That would work.

Hua Ai	Yes, the system is for drug screening and also disease modeling. So I think maybe previously not only physiologically maybe also pathological.
Kam Leong	Physiologically relevant meaning just to have a flow there. A physiological system.
Hanry Yu	You cannot add precision medicine before drug screening and disease modeling. Otherwise the other non-precision medicine types of the drug screening and disease modeling are excluded. So you should remove that.
Kam Leong	I think the definition right now is concise enough as well as descriptive. I think this is the best description.

(d) Final Definition and Voting for "Microphysiological System"

Microphysiological System

Interconnected tissues- or organs-on-a-chip using human cells to support physiologically-relevant evaluations of complex interacting biological systems for drug screening and disease modeling

Voting Yes	45
Voting No	1
Abstain	0
Total Votes	46
Number voting Yes or No	46
Percentage Yes Votes	97.8%

The definition achieved Consensus, having more than 75% Yes votes, with absolute number greater than 30.

D Organoid

(a) Possible Definitions of "Organoid" Included in Final Program

Self-organized three-dimensional tissue cultures that are typically derived from stem cells and replicate key functionality and biological complexity of an organ

(b) Kristi Anseth; Perspectives on "Organoid" and Suggested Definition

Kristi Anseth	The next term we have selected to discuss; lots of devices and organs on a chip are more top down engineered approaches. There is a complementary field that is more defined, the organoid, where we are developing organoid systems typically from single cells. They self-assemble to form complex structures. The idea here is defining an "organoid" as a "self-organized three-dimensional

tissue that are typically derived from stem cells and replicate key functionality and biological complexity of an organ." For those of you that aren't in the field you take a single, usually adult, progenitor cell, or it can be another stem cell, and from that single cell it grows, proliferates into colonies and differentiates to form multiple cell types and multiple features of an organ. It is a miniaturized version of an organ.

(c) Edited Discussion of "Organoid"

Andrés García	Kristi, this definition is very accurate for one community. I have also heard, for example, gut organoids from adult intestines. The gut crypts are also called organoids by that other community. I don't know if this is a case that you want to have two definitions. That one that you have there for stem cells is very accurate, but it doesn't capture the ones from an adult organoid.
Kam Leong	But the word typical captures that, no?
Andrés García	It is just they are very different. It is basically two different communities talking about different things. Since we work in this space and actually interact with people from both communities and there is always some confusion.
Kristin Anseth	I am not sure I understood your question. Are you saying that they isolate a portion of the crypt and grow that, instead of going from the single cell?
Andrés García	Yes, for the gut ones. Go to an adult organism, isolate the functional crypt unit. And if you put that in vitro will also form an organ and there is a community that calls that "organoids."
Hanry Yu	Yes, I agree with Andrés' comments. Because they are starting from the original mammary gland epithelial cells all the way involving adult cells, not stem cells or even progenitor cells. But it is sort of worthless as to think of this stem cell-based.
Kristin Anseth	And it is called an adult intestinal stem cell.
Hanry Yu	Yes. Whereas many people working with clinical setting actually isolate different cells from bodies, and primary cells, to do these organoid things.
Kristi Anseth	I see, thanks.
Kam Leong	Yes, because there could be cases of co-culturing hepatocytes with endothelial cells and forming tissue.
Arthur Coury	In every other case where I think there have been biomaterials involved in either containing or in channeling or delivering. Are, in some way, biomaterials going to be required or related to organoids?
Kristi Anseth	Yes, the answer is that is true. They are grown in Matrigel. And they are looking for alternative biomaterial systems because

	Matrigel is flawed for the clinical translation. So almost all of them use a biomaterial to grow them. Not all but almost.
Mario Barbosa	I think there is a concept missing there, which is the concept of tissue or the extracellular matrix. Because some organoids have extracellular matrix of the tissue incorporated in them, not just cells.
Kam Leong	Okay, but ECM is secreted by the cells too.
Carl Simon	My comments might also address that. In replicating key functionality and anatomy, I will also say because when I think of the organoids, even that picture you have there on the bottom left, it shows all those different morphologies that they grow into. So anatomically they resemble the organ. So key is anatomical.
Kristi Anseth	But I am missing the matrix part. I missed that.
Kam Leong	Typically derived from stem cells. Involving something.
Kristi Anseth	Yes.
Andrés García	Kristi I have a wordsmithing recommendation. I would probably say self-organized three-dimensional tissues that are derived from pluripotent stem cells or adults stem cells. Embedded within a matrix. Or a biomaterial if we want.
Kam Leong	But it does not need to be. If you see totally cell-based, you can also form an organ.
Kam Leong	Yes, right. Typically, sure.
Brendan Harley	So I had maybe one other wordsmith thing. Instead of anatomy we could talk about, because to get at the structural complexity because that could correspond to both organization but also cell-secreted ECM.
Kam Leong	That is "functional" not "functionality." Sounds good? Any other comments?
Hanry Yu	The stem cell doesn't have to be adult stem cell, it can be primary cells. There's a large community of people doing this.
Kam Leong	From pluripotent or adult cells.
Kai Zhang	They're just cells?
Kam Leong	Just cells.
Peter Ma	We are listing all types of cells.
Kam Leong	Well … Stem cells are really, yes. Yes, you seen pluripotent stem cells.
Kristi Anseth	Andrés, are you okay if I take out "pluripotent"?
Andrés García	Yes, rather than that wording. I think stem cells would be better than just cells.
Xiaobing Fu	My suggestion is that "stem cell" is enough, because stem cell includes pluripotent and other cells, they have ability to regenerate the tissue. So if you use many stem cells. It is not necessary. Just stem cells is enough.

Kam Leong	Okay.
Andrés García	I think "replicate" is too strong. I think some biologists may disagree with that; maybe "model" or "recapitulate."
Kam Leong	Recapitulate. That sounds good.
Rena Bizios	Stem cells or primary cells, in proposed stem or primary cells. Take out one cells. Delete one of the cells, yes. And that recapitulate for me, I preferred the replicate. Because it indicates some kind of imitation or duplication or something that we are doing in vitro to duplicate the biological or physiological situation.
Kam Leong	That syntax would probably mean different things to different people.
Rena Bizios	I would change "recapitulate" to "mimic."
Kam Leong	That's another choice, but okay.
Andrés García	I would just leave it at stem cells.
Kam Leong	No, but you could use adult cells to form this organoid. So, is everyone happy with mimic, replicate, or recapitulate? I mean they are very similar. Any preference? Any strong preference? Okay. Are you all right with that, mimic? Bill, final comment.
William Wagner	I just noted that at the beginning, it is typically derived from stem cells. And I think that was better than everything that we went around, because it is "typically."
Kristi Anseth	I know, I'm trying to get rid of two "typicals."
William Wagner	Yes, just move the one of there. And then take the other one out. You could say "typically derived from stem cells and embedded in a matrix." Because the typically could apply to both.
Kam Leong	Right.

(d) Final Definition and Voting for "Organoid"

Organoid

Self-organized three-dimensional tissues that are typically derived from stem cells, and embedded in a matrix, and mimic key functional, structural and biological complexity of an organ

Voting Yes	45
Voting No	2
Abstain	0
Total Votes	47
Number voting Yes or No	47
Percentage Yes Votes	95.7%

The definition achieved Consensus, having more than 75% Yes votes, with absolute number greater than 30.

(e) Further Commentary on the Definition of "Organoid"

In the context that David Williams was given the authority to make minor grammatical alterations, a slightly better wording is as follows; it is this which is confirmed to have consensus:

Organoid

Self-organized three-dimensional tissues that are typically derived from stem cells, and embedded in a matrix, and which mimic the key functional, structural and biological complexity of an organ

E Biomaterials Genome/Biomaterialomics

(a) Possible Definitions of "Biomaterials Genome" Included in Final Program

Integration of computational tools, databases and experimental techniques to accelerate the discovery and design of novel biomaterials and their integration into medical devices

(b) Kristi Anseth; Perspectives on "Biomaterials Genome" and Suggested Definition

Kristi Anseth   Next were going to move on to some of the themes about contemporary areas related to biomaterial chemistry and so I clustered some of the topics in the pre-reading material that relate to more commonly used terms now of precision biomaterials, biomaterials genome and bioclick reactions. And then adaptive biomaterials. Depending on how the discussion goes we will likely vote on all of these. So the first, and we have already had some of this discussion, is "precision biomaterials," a term that is starting to be used more, meaning in some senses some people would call this personalized biomaterials. But I think precision biomaterials is a little bit more contemporary now. And the idea here is to show that we no longer think of a single biomaterial integrated into a device being used to treat all patients but on a spectrum. How you design biomaterials that are capable to interact very specifically with the biology of a patient.

Kristi Anseth   A single patient or a set of patients. Maybe they all have breast cancer to elicit desired predictable and personalized outcomes. So that's one general definition. The other focuses on what it means to have a precision biomaterial. And that means you "customize material chemistry, or device fabrication." Integrating specific bioactive components. "And/or incorporating patient data analysis to detect or treat disease or injury in a specific patient or subset of patients." So the second one is a little bit more clunky but it brings in a little bit more of the biomaterial science. The first one I think is one that's a little bit more concise and is the intent of what a precision biomaterial would do. So maybe we could do a first consensus how many people would like to discuss this as one of the terms that we would define? No-one. Okay.

Kristi Anseth   I'm just wondering if we should spend time on the term precision biomaterial. We've already defined biomaterial, no. No. Okay.

Kristi Anseth   Then we'll move on. Second one is "biomaterials genome." We hear a lot about the "materials genome" and many people don't know what the materials genome is even though it has been around for probably almost a decade now. The idea of that term and how it applies to biomaterials is really just about "integrating computational tools, data sets and experimental techniques designed towards accelerating, discovering design of new biomaterials and their integration into medical devices." It is just a way of analyzing and integrating machine learning computational tools to accelerate the process of materials discovery. So, how many people would like to integrate this into the biomaterials community as a definition? Okay. So let's spend some time talking about this one.

(c) Edited Discussion of "Biomaterials Genome and Related Terms"

Maria J. Vicent   There were a few papers a few years ago talking about polymer genomics, so maybe genomics is better than genome.

Kam Leong   Also, is there a reason to emphasize the integration into medical devices? Or we could just stop there and cut out the last phrase.

Rena Bizios   I think that we should keep the last phrase.

Cato Laurencin   I have always had concerns about this because the term has nothing to do with genomics. It is the only term I have ever seen that talks about something that has nothing to do with something, right? So it is a definition. I mean the concept is sort of good on a scale one level where you say OK I am going to do something and try to create a revolution, just like the genomics revolution, we are going to do what they did in genomics, but do it for materials. That is sort of the whole concept between the material genomics initiative to do something in materials that you did in genomics. But it has nothing to do with genomics in terms of the science of it so it is a very confusing term.

Rui Reis   I agree with Cato I think this is really the case there are people in Europe that are calling this "materiomics" or "biomateriomics" as you prefer because this is really nothing to do what genomics.

Maria J. Vicent   Because it's not only genomics I will agree with that, so I will put "omics" in general.

John Brash   It is "biomaterialomics."

Joachim Kohn   We actually have written a paper stepping into the "omics" area, and omics is the idea of this large datasets. This is in line with Maria, what you said. So this is about opportunities and challenges for biomaterial science and engineering. And the transition of the field into large datasets and so that fits into here, and Cato is also correct, of course. Genomics is the wrong term for it. The "omics" is what we are interested in, so "materiomics" is used in Europe a lot, and so perhaps we can change the genomics to "materialomics," that would be in line with the European use of the term.

Joachim Kohn   And then the definition is quite accurate actually. It's the integration of computational tools, databases, big data, and experimental techniques to accelerate the discovery and design of new biomaterials. I am not sure that it is necessary to integrate them into medical devices, I have not seen that explicitly in some of the papers.

Timmie Topoleski   I just was recalling yesterday, it is a small thing that we talked about essentially banning the term "novel" from biomaterials, right? Can we make it new biomaterials?

Kam Leong   Okay.

Timmie Topoleski   Or emerging biomaterials?

Kam Leong   I agree with Joachim's point, I thought this is David's view for this kind of meeting. Define a new term that is unique to our field. This is a good opportunity.

Xingdong Zhang   What is a materials genome? It is not clear. I think the biomaterials genome is an elemental fact of the biomaterials. The element fact is a materials gene. So why not explain the difference of materials gene and the human gene.

Kai Zhang   It is going to be hard though because there are two major projects now in China on the biomaterials genome initiative, and Professor Xingdong Zhang is the one who designed the projects. Professor Zhang just mentioned, in order to define the biomaterials genome, first we need to know what are the biomaterials genes? And he thinks biomaterials genes are the characteristics of the biomaterial.

Kam Leong   So those are the basic elements?

Kai Zhang   Basically the element decides the materials structure. So it's important.

Kam Leong   I think that is what other people use for the building unit of materials, but this topic is going to impact our field in the near future, and I think it would be nice to come up with a term. We all agree that genomics is not a good term, so if we could come up with another term with all the brain power in this room.

Jiandong Ding   I think that according to the comments of Professor Zhang we can modify the first item. For instance, the integration of computational tools, large databases, experimental techniques to explore the material elements and combine them to discover and design a new material.

Kam Leong	That is good, but we still need to come up with a term.
Joachim Kohn	Please remember that we have viruses in our computer now, and it is a sign for the importance of biology to our time that we are using biological terms in unrelated disciplines now. The idea to speak about materials genes is just like when you are speaking about computer viruses, it is kind of like an adaptation. Now there is really a fundamental question whether you want to endorse that sloppy language, or whether you want to come back and actually say materials do not have genes, only living organisms have genes. And what we are really speaking about is traits or characteristics. And on the other hand, you could go with the flow of the majority and just accept the language. I think this should be a vote.
Kam Leong	Yes.
Joachim Kohn	And then we can go from there.
Kam Leong	Let us come back to that.
Jian Ji	I think we can use the genomics because I think if we only use the "omics" it is something greater, but what we do for the material genomics is we want to find the basic material environment for that. I think we can keep this, because genome does not exactly mean the DNA. It's just the basic element for the biological sex. So it is the same for the material science.
Xingdong Zhang	I would like to speak again. The biomaterial gene is a basic element of biomaterials. And the materials gene is materials basic element, which decided the materials structure and properties.
Kam Leong	Right. So I think you like the phrase there. The basic materials elements.
Xingdong Zhang	Yes. Yes.
Maria J. Vicent	For the definition I would delete "for medical devices," because they could also apply to applications that are not devices. I would delete that.
Kam Leong	Delete that last phrase, okay.
Arthur Coury	In the original definition of a biomaterial it was always affiliated with a medical device, and that was accepted. In our current definition, we avoid the term medical device and so I was actually going to also suggest medical product, I am sorry to see that go, actually. For example, Matrigel, we would probably consider that a biomaterial, by the definition, but it is not considered a medical device, it is at least called a biologic by the FDA's definition. I would say medical products rather than medical device.
Kam Leong	Okay.
Rena Bizios	Listen to the discussion, what we have here is something, I do not have a title, but I distill this information. What we are talking

about are the biomaterials in the genomics era. And it is of course the future, but it doesn't become a title for a definition. But that is what we're trying to do. What will biomaterials be, or what they will, they should be in this era, the biological world, the physiological world is moving in that particular direction. Can we come up with a term that reflects that?

Yuliang Zhao   To avoid the statement about the meaning of the word, I have another suggestion. Perhaps we could use another way to define this term, for example. So the biomaterials genomics we can say that these are application of the material genomics in biomaterials. That is simple and a very clear and include all these ideas.

Kam Leong   Wait, I couldn't get what you mean.

Yuliang Zhao   So apply the theory and technology of the material genomics in biomaterials.

Kam Leong   That is too long.

Yuliang Zhao   It is not. It is much shorter than this one.

Kam Leong   Not the definition, I was just saying about the term that we would like.

Yuliang Zhao   That is not term, that is the definition. What I say is the definition. You can use the term "biomaterial genomics," so for the definition is appropriate you can use this, this is another way.

Kam Leong   The definition.

Yuliang Zhao   So the definition is applying the theory and technology of the material genomics in biomaterials.

Kam Leong   Right.

Yuliang Zhao   And you can put a note into it to get the definition of the "materials genomics."

Kam Leong   But I thought the major dispute right now is to use the word "genomics" or not.

Jui-Che Lin   Regarding the name of this term, I check the biological field, they say genomics, or genome proteomics, metabolomics so anything ends with the O-M-E, in a sense we are trying to define the term, saying we are using a lot of, I am okay with the definition one, but if according to the biologists they probably would name this term ends with O-M-E. "Biomateriome," we are creating a new term.

Kam Leong   That is okay. That is another choice. Yes, please.

Mário Barbosa   The origin of the name is Greek, so we have some Greek colleagues here who can perhaps help us in deciding in the original meaning of the name. Biologists start talking about genes and genomes. It was a Greek word, genus, I think. And what is the meaning of that word in Greek?

Kam Leong   Origin is it? No?

Rena Bizios	Yes, is very basic situation you would say origin, yes, it is the closest definition.
Carl Simon	So, by analogy to the genes for materials, what I'm seeing online is that it comes back to properties, so you may want to have the word properties, I think the word "properties" has to be in there, because magnetic properties, or how it performs under stress, or those sorts of things. Diffusion. So basic material properties, from what I'm reading about materials genome and materials genome initiative, it comes back to starting with the genes and the genes are the properties. So measuring properties of materials and using that to do the modeling.
Kai Zhang	I will try to be concise. Number one, from the name while we are inventing some new terms we need to be respectful to what already being in the field. So there is already the materials genome initiative. Both in China and in the United States. And government funding agencies, they support it so much. I am not against inventing a new term, but if you do not have a better term, we would rather just keep as the biomaterials genome, that is my personal perspective.
Kai Zhang	I am going to translate Professor Zhang's idea regarding the definition of biomaterial genome. He thinks that biomaterials genome is the combination of the genes of biomaterials. Let me see. The genes of the biomaterials are the fundamental factors of materials which will determine the structure and properties of biomaterials.
Kam Leong	Okay, the definition seems to me a little bit easier to settle. Last. David, please. Thanks.
David Williams	Thank you Kam. I agree with most of what you said, I think it's very important that we get this right, we introduce this as a new area. And I am quite happy with the first one of these. My real problem is the terms. I like the idea of "biomaterome." That's the only one I like. I don't like keeping the word "genome" in there, because it is, as we have seen, this has got nothing to do with genes. "Biomaterialomics" is a horrible word, and I would not like that to be in a dictionary. But biomaterome has a lot more going for it as far as I'm concerned. I would go along with that.
Kam Leong	I also like that term.
Brendan Harley	I would sort of follow on with that. I like the" biomaterialome," I will have to get used to saying it, but I think one of the other aspects is instead of just exploring basic material elements, we are really talking about defining the combinations.
Kam Leong	That is good, can be separate because we have to move on. Brendan, it is fine. Let us talk about the name first. The three choices. "Biomaterialome," "Biomaterials Genome," and

	"Biomaterial Genomics." Let us have a show of hands quickly on that first, and then we move on.
William Wagner	So the "ome," like "materialome" or "genome" refers to the collection of those properties, and the "omics" is the operation, that is my understanding. So the definition is the operation on the "genome," right? So it is "genomics." So it should be "ics," not "ome." As far as the terms have been used in terms of proteome - proteomics, genome - genomics.
Kam Leong	Biomaterialomics. So that's another choice. But should we keep the original one?
Nicholas Peppas	May I make a comment, one minute on what Bill just said. I know I have been quiet, because what we use in Greek is really not relevant anymore, because things have changed significantly. But what Bill said is correct. That the field that studies is "ics" in Greek. And it's not "ome," which is basically an entity that describes particular part of the body or of the cell, or whatever.
Nicholas Peppas	So, if you really insist upon using something that has the "om" in it, it should be "omics" rather than "ome," but again, as I said, things have moved further away from the Greek terms. That's why both Rena and I were quiet there.
Jian Ji	I think it is better we make a definition, people will be use it. If we create a totally new thing, I am just wondering who will use it. Of course, the people here will use it.
Kam Leong	That is right. At least the 50 people here. But since we have the thought leaders in the field.
Ki Dong Park	I think if we really want to create a biomaterials term, we need to think of using the whole materials science. Because, for example, material genome has been used in the materials field. If now we create a new "biomaterialomics," we may need to think if the people in the whole material science agree with the "materialomics."
Kam Leong	Right, so that is the mission in one way. We are going to use the computational tools, databases, and so on. Machine learning, and so on. Kristi, are you comfortable with the terms? So any objections to biomaterialomics? Yes. Then we refine the definition. The definition has been discussed a lot and I am guessing that you are happy. Kind of happy. Okay, let us vote.

(d) Final Definition and Voting for "Biomaterialomics"

Biomaterialomics

Integration of computational tools, large databases and experimental techniques to explore the basic material elements and combine them to discover and design new biomaterials for medical products

Voting Yes	36
Voting No	11
Abstain	1
Total Votes	48
Number voting Yes or No	47
Percentage Yes Votes	76.6%

The definition achieved Consensus, having more than 75% Yes votes, with absolute number greater than 30.

F Bio-click Reactions

(a) Possible Definitions of "Bio-click Reactions" Included in Final Program

1. Orthogonal reaction partners that react near biological conditions, produce non-toxic or no byproducts, yield single and stable products, and proceed quickly to high yield in a complex reaction milieu
2. Class of biocompatible small molecule reactions commonly used in bioconjugation of biomaterials with biologics, hydrogels and other biomaterials scaffolds, and bioseparation and biosensing reactions

(b) Kristi Anseth; Perspectives on "Bio-click Reactions" and Suggested Definition

Kristi Anseth	Okay, the next term in the material chemistry is one that has really emerged over the last five to ten years. And that is the concept of click reactions. So, I came up with a definition for bio-click reactions, those of you that aren't familiar, I just gave some examples, but it's an emerging area or concept where you have combinations, so usually two species that react orthogonally. They are very specific to one another, and they have partners, and for the bio-click they react near biological conditions that produce nontoxic or no byproducts, and they yield single and stable products, and proceed quite quickly to high yield in a complex reaction milieu.
Kristi Anseth	So I was proposing this reaction so we could give guidance as to what is a bio-click reaction when people start using this in the biomaterials community. That defines the reactions that can be classified this way. The second one is a little bit more on how they're used. So, it's a class of biocompatible, small molecule reactions commonly used in bioconjugation to biomaterials with biologics, synthesis of hydrogels and other biomaterial scaffolds. Or they are used for bioseparations, and biosensing reactions.

| Kristi Anseth | I am not sure that defines the bio-click as well, but it gives some insight into the uses. If we think this is an important term, I would vote for number one. So those of you that work in the chemistry. David? |

(c) Edited Discussion of "Bio-click Reactions"

David Williams	Yes, I agree with one. If you go for number two, you cannot use the word "biocompatible," that does not exist.
Kristi Anseth	Thank you. I respectfully accept that. That slipped by. Thank you.
Kam Leong	So, is there any other comments?
Arthur Coury	I am not sure that the whole organic polymer chemistry conjugation community agrees that all those reactions are click. I mean what is it, the azide reaction.
Kristi Anseth	So my list on the right, the top one with the copper, most people would say that is not bio-click. All the ones below it, it is a growing list. Those of you who work in the field, I just thought it might be useful to give some guidance. But, Art, are we missing some terms that you think we should include?
Arthur Coury	Well, I just think we might create controversy over what a click reaction is if we use all of those. I know there is a commonly used term for click reaction. It is almost an addition reaction. I am not sure it is that important a term to address actually.
Kristi Anseth	Okay. We don't have to address it, but I am not sure I said it was an addition reaction, right? Well, I guess that is a question for the group. Especially those of you that I think work on synthesis of materials, do we think this is an important term that we want to define for the community? Maybe just a show of hands? I suggested this one, so I am raising mine, but I am fine if other people don't want to. And those that know about the field and feel strongly that we shouldn't? Okay. Maybe we could just spend a short amount of time, see if we have some consensus.
Nicholas Peppas	I think the term is important. I think many new biomaterials are being prepared by this, and frankly this is one case where I will say Kristi's probably, you and the other Kristi at Delaware, click, are probably the world's leaders in the use of this technology in the biomedical field. So I will accept your definition as set here. Thanks.
Kam Leong	Thanks. That's helpful. Any other comments? Joachim.
Joachim Kohn	I would like to point out that click reactions are actually very well defined in chemistry. Every organic chemist knows what they are. I am not 100 percent sure that it's necessary to define them here, not because they are not important, but because it's well established technology and we are teaching it in second grade organic chemistry. And so, not everything that is widely used and well understood requires a new definition. That's my opinion. I want to

	point out that I am not opposed to it in anyway. I just wanted to point out that I see limited use for spending a lot of time on making up a new definition.
Kam Leong	But for the future, I think more and more of us will use this bio-click, and this is a new definition, and so if it is a little bit different from click, I think it is good. David.
David Williams	I think it is important to include it. You have got most aspects in that definition, but the grammar and syntax seem to be totally wrong. The term is" bio-click reactions," and you start with "orthogonal reaction partners." That's not consistent as far as I can see. And the phrase," produce non-toxic or no by-products," I think that could be phrased a little bit differently.
Kam Leong	Okay, while that is being edited, any other comments?
John Brash	I think this is a very good definition. I would like to have clarification on the word "orthogonal" in this context.
Kam Leong	All right.
Kristi Anseth	The idea would be that they have a complementing reaction, or that they are specific so that if you mixed together four of these pairs, these two would find each other, and these two would find each other, and you wouldn't get cross-products. They are orthogonal, the reaction.
David Williams	Sorry, Kam can you just go back, I am not sure I understand the syntax of that first sentence. We are talking about reactions, not groups, aren't we? Or are they processes? So could that include processes involving orthogonal etc.?
Kam Leong	Chemical reactions.
Kristi Anseth	I am using reactions a lot.
Kam Leong	Right.
Arthur Coury	If you are expanding the understanding of the word click, I mean click is used all the time in terms of a specific reaction. If you are reacting an N-hydroxysuccinimide with an amine or with a thiol, to me that has never been called a click reaction, and now it is, and maybe it will be accepted, maybe not, but I think it could create a controversy.
Kam Leong	But it is a new term, bio-click is the first-generation definition of this term, I think it is good. I like what Nick said, Kristi is one of the few world leaders. Let us not dwell too much time on the refinement of the language, can we give the command to David later on to really refine it, then we move on vote. Laura please.
Laura Poole-Warren	Yes Kristi, perhaps instead of "orthogonal," you could use "complementary" or something like that? Would that work?
Kristi Anseth	Yes, I think I can. I think "orthogonal" is just what the chemists use, so that is why I would put it in, but yes.

(d) Final Definition and Voting for "Bio-click Reactions"

Bio-click Reactions

Processes involving complementary functional groups that react near biological conditions, produce non-toxic or no byproducts, yield single and stable products, and proceed quickly to high yield in a complex reaction milieu

Voting Yes	30
Voting No	12
Abstain	2
Total Votes	45
Number voting Yes or No	42
Percentage Yes Votes	71.4%

The definition achieved Provisional Consensus, having more than 50% Yes votes.

(e) Further Commentary on the Definition of "Bio-click Reactions"

In the context that David Williams was given the authority to make minor grammatical alterations, a slightly better wording has been considered; indeed, the delegates suggested that some adjustment would be appropriate, especially concerning "orthogonal." The revised definition given below was confirmed after the conference.

Bio-click Reactions

Processes involving orthogonal groups that react under near-biological conditions, yielding single, stable products, with either no or non-toxic byproducts, proceeding quickly in complex milieu, with high yield

G Bioink

(a) Possible Definitions of "Bioink" Included in Final Program

1. Biomaterials that can be extruded and otherwise integrated into additive manufacturing processes to print 3D structures

2. Materials used in printing of scaffolds that mimic the extracellular matrix environment and support the adhesion, proliferation and differentiation of living cells

(b) Kristi Anseth; Perspectives on "Bioink" and Suggested Definition

Kristi Anseth	The definitions that I came up with for bioinks were first, "a biomaterial that can be extruded or otherwise integrated into additive manufacturing processes to print 3D structures." And then the second was "materials used in printing of scaffolds that mimic the extra-cellular matrix environment and support the adhesion proliferation and differentiation of living cells."

| Kristi Anseth | Not sure I love either of them, they are not quite perfect. We need to wordsmith some of them, but the second one is focusing more on what you would put into a bioink, and the first one is focusing on the properties of material that allow it to be integrated into additive manufacturing. |

(c) Edited Discussion of "Bioink"

Rena Bizios	I prefer the second because otherwise it is an ink, and people have used it for everything from toys to all kinds of non-biological things. It makes it "bio" when we bring in the cells and we maintain their viability and functionality. If we put them in there and they are not functional, they are not viable, it is the end of the story. The other one is a more general, I agree, but for me the second one is more close to the biomaterial-related application.
Wei Sun	In the biofabrication field, we have very short understanding definition for "bioink." We call that as a cell delivery medium because it may not be just printing a scaffold, and it may not just integrate and assemble cell. They may have all this function, or they may have only one function, but I think with "bioink," the major rule of bioink is to deliver cells. I prefer to consider that as a cell delivery medium.
Arthur Coury	I was going to ask the same question, what do you call a printing press that delivers a cell and its matrix, or a cell and a hydrogel into a form that you desire to have? I used to think that was bioink, but this does not incorporate cells in it.
Kam Leong	The second part, yes please.
John Ramshaw	Going back to that comment, if it's just to deliver cells, there's people doing coaxial printing with both components considered as bioinks, if only one of them is there to produce the cell delivery and the others is a protection against well the UV light or whatever else is used to cure the system? So I am unclear that it has to be cells, because I think that those protective layers would still be called inks.
Andrés García	I do not think the second definition captures all the activity in this area. For example, the instances that you are putting cells within materials where there is no adhesion of the cell to that material like a chondrocyte. Similarly, why does it have to mimic the extracellular matrix? You could make a material that has no characteristic of the extracellular matrix and it is still used to print the cells or the analog of the tissue.
Rena Bizios	I agree with Andrés' comment, we do not have necessarily to mimic, but we have to provide that extracellular matrix otherwise the cells are not going to make it. So the word, if I understood correctly, your comment pertains to the choice of the word "mimic"? Can we come up with a different word? What we have to explain that this, whatever the process is, the material provides the equivalent of an extra cellular matrix for the cells.

Andrés García	So the senses that the cell does not adhere or interact with the medium, so the rest of the statement that says supports the adhesion probably function and differentiation of living cells may not be accurate in all cases.
Rena Bizios	We can modify that along the lines to support survival and function of living cells. We can modify them, I am not against this.
Joachim Kohn	I think the first definition is especially sweet and accurate and short and I like it a lot. We do a lot of 3D printing, and we 3D print metals and other electronic parts, and so bioinks is everything that is used in the 3D printing in a medical or tissue engineering or regeneration application. So biomaterials, that is captured in the fact that we say biomaterials. It is not automotive metals, it is not other things. And that they can be extruded. And the only thing that I would like to add is that it doesn't have to contain cells. I think some people said that it doesn't have to contain cells and it is still bioprinting, it is still bioink, but it may contain cells.
Kam Leong	That is a major point, we have to come back to that.
Elizabeth Cosgriff-H	I think I would have to disagree, and I would defer to Wei Sun, I mean he has the Biofabrication journal so I am sure he sees most of this field coming through there. I think bioinks and bioprinting refers to printing with cells. People may be using it differently, but I think we have to be very careful if we are going to define something that is different than something established in the field.
Helen Lu	I think along the same lines, I was just curious that if you are printing growth factors, is that a bioink? You know if you print something that maintains bioactivity of either the cell or the factor that is being printed, I consider that a bioink. If you are printing just polymer that is not necessarily alive or has bioactivity in the sense of being a biological species, I would not consider that a bioink.
Rui Reis	I think we can bioprint things that are not 3D, so 3D should not be in there for sure because you can print membranes, you can print just cells for a screening system or whatever so I don't think this really should be in there. And I completely agree that we don't need to have the ECM properties in there because you can print things that are not for cell adhesion and there is no ECM whatsoever, the idea is just to support the cells in some way.
Xiaobing Fu	Maybe we can use very short sentences. Bioink is a material with different function, and they use the ink in 3D printing. It's enough.
Wei Sun	First of all, I would like to say the bioink is with cells. Without cells, we don't call that bioink because we can call that biomaterial, that's number one. Number two, I would like this definition to be more inclusive. That is why I do not suggest putting scaffold in, put 3D or extruding, because those are very specific. Because we can always find different cases in which a bioink is applied but is not for scaffold, is not

	being extruded. For example, inkjet, even if it is not for 3D machine because people do print cells. That is why I would like to see, that it is nothing but a cell delivery medium. Because when you talk about the function, when we deliver this medium and you know we know that this is ink, the material will transfer a cell, protect a cell, or position a cell. But this not always the case because you can always find individual cases which they don't serve that function. But if you want a definition to be more generic, so I do rather to have a short phrase.
Rena Bizios	Short is good but it has to be describing the essential elements, which makes this "bio," and I go back to something that Helen said, which is to expand a little bit from the cells to include bioactive chemical compounds, because sometimes you add growth factors in addition to cells, or growth factors and some other chemical compounds. I think that is how I understood Helen's comment.
Wei Sun	I understand what you thought, but in reality this may not be the case. Let me give an example. If you print alginate, the function is not bioactivity. Alginate is to keep cell survival but provides for the structure stability. But if you add the gelatin, if you add fibronectin, then you make a different bioink, then they are adding bioactivity. But you cannot say gelatin or alginate is not a bioink because alginate mixed with cell is very standard, popular bioink. So that is why sometimes, without more specification, it may be better.
Rena Bizios	I think in order to resolve this particular comment here, I will go back to something that David had mentioned for another definition - it may contain cells and/or bioactive components and that covers everything. Sometimes you have the cell, sometimes you have the compound, and sometimes you don't have anything. So is that the solution to this? Structures which may contain "cells and/or bioactive components"?
Kam Leong	But the important point here is not and/or. My understanding is that bioink must have cells.
Kristi Anseth	So if we want, regarding Helen's point, if we wanted to expand the definition into a new area saying that these inks that also contain bioactive components, we just have to understand that that would be a new definition that is not accepted yet. So it would be forward looking.
Maria J. Vicent	We just make it simpler and in the third definition, we just put something like cell delivery biomaterial based medium. So with biomaterial based you can include those bioactive items. And there are cells which are the main component, not the biomaterial.
Peter Ma	I think cell medium keeps cell alive. Probably we are thinking similar ideas in there. But one thing I think really need to be included is for printing. If you do not have printing, we should not call it an ink. It's just media. No polymer, it is a cell-containing media. That is not

	printable. Just as regular cell growth media, there is no polymer whatsoever. Therefore, we have to say for printing. Without "for printing," it is not an ink.
Elizabeth Cosgriff-H	Maybe for the first one, "cell laden biomaterials "or something along that line.
Brendan Harley	I was going to add something similar in this, I actually like the last one in some ways. Cell delivery, bio, you know the thing about an ink is that it has, we can agree, it has got an element that would have cells in it, and but the other half of it is, it maybe does not have to be printed but there is some structure or some design or something that you can do with it. I think that something along the lines of, it does not have to be printed but that you can be, it can then have a structure created from it or patterned with, something along those, some of those words I think are the key differentiation between my cell culture medium with my cells in it that would not be a bioink.
Kam Leong	That's a key point. Bill, are you happy with it?
William Wagner	Yes it, I think it is clear we are hearing that there is already a term that is pretty well accepted in that community that cells have to be there, and if we do another one we just have multiple definitions.
Kam Leong	Then the other point is whether it has to be printed. That I would like to just have defined or discussion. I personally feel that it should be. Please, you are the editor-in-chief of the journal.
Wei Sun	Then we can add a few, for example we call that it does this cell delivery medium for 3D printing. The reason I did not say that is because we don't even talk about bioprinting, so then you get into another chaos talking about this new definition. If a 3D bioprinting, that probably enough.
Kam Leong	Okay, so for 3D bioprinting.
Rena Bizios	If you are using cells, my mind will go to the liquid in which we culture the cells, so that particular term could cause more confusion than it will help. So the word medium should not be there. You can call it biomaterial-based carrier or something else, but not medium.
Kam Leong	So let's have a final focus on the best definition.
Kristi Anseth	Which one should we focus on, one or two?
Kam Leong	But I thought the "cell-laden biomaterial" is a good term to cover a lot of things. And then "3D bioprinting" should be there, maybe in the first definition.
Kristi Anseth	But don't I have to print?
Kam Leong	For, maybe for 3D bioprinting. But is a little bit redundant, right? Bioprinting is already meaning printing cells, isn't it? No?
Wei Sun	Maybe let's think it this way, we have HP printer printing with normal paper. Then we have ink. How we define that ink? That ink is nothing but you know prepared, used for that HP printer, right? So I

	think it is okay. If you have "cell-laden biomaterial for…" you don't even say 3D, maybe for bioprinting. Maybe even better, because that not exclude for the 2D, some people do print in 2D.
Kam Leong	So you are suggesting cell-laden biomaterials?
Wei Sun	Cell-laden biomaterials for bioprinting.
Kam Leong	For bioprinting.
Wei Sun	Or you want to say even for printing. Maybe for bioprinting better.
Kam Leong	Please, for bioprinting yes.
Deon Bezuidenhout	I have a question whether the carrier is the ink, or whether the carrier plus the cells is the ink. Which defines the ink?
Kam Leong	Combination.
David Williams	I think number one gives you everything. I am slightly concerned about number two, which refers to printing of scaffolds as the first part of that, which I don't particularly like.
William Wagner	I think it is a minor point, but I think we should be singular. I don't know why we would be plural here and not in other areas.
Nicholas Peppas	I would like to suggest that colleagues consider a little bit more one, for the simple reason that almost everybody who uses the word bioink uses it in relation to printing and uses it in relation to the ability to create filaments that can be used in artificial organs. So there is the embedded idea that whether it's 2D or 3D printing, that should be somehow mentioned. For example, a hydrogel with cells in it, and you give it out within a syringe, and you push the cells out like this. Is that a bioink? No. So, there has to be something relative that printing ability.
Kam Leong	Right. Because with one we do not have to worry about the definition of bioprinting, so that could be independent. So shall we go with one and then we go with the voting please.

(d) Final Definition and Voting for "Bioink"

Bioink

Cell-laden biomaterial that can be integrated into additive manufacturing processes to print 2D and 3D structures

Voting Yes	41
Voting No	5
Abstain	2
Total Votes	48
Number voting Yes or No	46
Percentage Yes Votes	89.1%

The definition achieved Consensus, having more than 75% Yes votes, with absolute number greater than 30.

H Other Biomaterials-Based Biotechnology Terms: No Voting, With or Without Discussion

A number of other terms were scheduled for discussion and voting during Session VI but time allowed for only limited discussion and no votes were taken. The definitions proposed by the Plenary Speaker are included here for completeness.

Microfluidics

1. The behavior, control and manipulation of fluids that are geometrically constrained to small, typically sub-millimeter, scale
2. The science of manipulating and controlling fluids, usually in the range of microliters to picoliters in networks of channels with dimensions from tens to hundreds of micrometers
3. The technology of manufacturing microminiaturized devices containing chambers, channels, and unit operations through which fluids flow in a controlled manner

Point-of-care Devices

1. Devices used to obtain diagnostic results while with the patient or close to the patient
2. Simple medical tests that can be performed at the bedside or in remote locations near the patient

Biosensor

1. A device used to detect the presence or concentration of a biological analyte
2. A device that uses a living organism or biological molecules, especially enzymes or antibodies, to detect the presence of chemicals

Regenerative Biology

Studying, mimicking, or engineering the processes by which organisms replace or restore injured or amputated tissues and organs

Bioprinting

1. The use of 3D additive manufacturing technology that typically incorporates one or more biological components, viable cells, growth factors, and/or bioactive materials
2. The use of 3D manufacturing technologies combined with bioinks and viable cells to recreate desired tissues or organ

Biofabrication

The production of complex living and non-living biological products from raw materials such as living cells, molecules, extracellular matrices, and biomaterials

Precision Biomaterials

1. Biomaterials capable of interacting with the biology of a patient or set of patients to elicit desired, predictable and personalized outcomes

2. Customized material chemistry, device fabrication, bioactive components, and/or patient data analysis to detect or treat disease or injury in a specific patient or subsets of patients

Adaptive Biomaterials

1. Active biomaterials that can change their functional properties, typically without degradation, in response to an external stimulus
2. Well-defined and functionalized polymers that are responsive to desired physiological processes
3. Examples: covalent adaptable networks, self-healing biomaterials

Bioimaging

1. The imaging of biological materials, structures, systems or processes
2. Methods that non-invasively visualize biological structures
3. The production of images of living organisms by X-rays, ultrasound, magnetic resonance imaging, light, electrons

Functional Imaging

1. Imaging modalities directed at the evaluation of activity and function of cells, tissues or organs
2. Imaging techniques that detect or measure changes in physiological processes, including metabolism, blood flow, and local biochemical compositions, etc.

Surface Topography

Delineation of the natural and artificial features of a surface from a flat plane

Surface Patterning

The deliberate, regular and spatially-controlled modification of surfaces through physical, chemical or biological means in order to enhance specific properties and performance

Immunomodulation

1. Modification of the immune response or the functioning of the immune system by the action of a biomaterial or other biomacromolecule
2. Adjustment of the immune response to a desired level

Immunoengineering

The application of engineering tools and principles to
1. quantitatively study the immune system in health and disease
2. develop new therapies or improve existing therapies by enhancing, suppressing or modulating the immune responses

Materiobiology

Editor's Note: One of the delegates, Changsheng Liu, asked that consideration be given to the term "Materiobiology," which he had recently introduced in a paper in Chemical Reviews,[1] and which he defined as:

> A scientific interdiscipline that studies the biological effects of the properties of biomaterials on biological functions at cell, tissue, organ, and the whole organism levels, discloses the relationships between the characteristics of materials and the features of biology

The topic was discussed very briefly in the last session, but it was decided that it was too premature to include this concept at this time, and no attempt was made to modify or vote on the definition.

I Nanoscale and Nanotechnology

The nanoscale figures prominently in many biomaterials contexts. It was not specifically discussed in relation to any specific biomaterials definitions, but there was significant contribution to the understanding of the nanoscale in biological environments.

David Williams defined the nanoscale in the introductory comments to the conference and these Proceedings as follows:

Nanoscale

Having one or more dimensions of the order of 100 nm or less

He further defined other nano-based words in the preliminary papers for Session I, as follows:

Nanotechnology

The design, characterization, production and application of structures, devices and systems by controlling shape and size at the nanoscale

Nanomaterial

Material with one or more external dimensions, or an internal structure, which could exhibit novel characteristics compared to the same material without nanoscale features

Nanoparticle

Particle with one or more dimensions at the nanoscale
Note that the alternative is "Particle with two or more dimensions at the nanoscale"

In preliminary papers for Session V, Nicholas Peppas used the following definitions:

---

[1] Li Y, Xiao Y, Liu C, The horizon of materiobiology: A perspective on material-guided cell behaviors and tissue engineering, *Chem Rev* 2017;117:4376-421.

Nanoparticles

Particles at the sub-micron scale

Nanotechnology

The science of manipulating materials at the sub-micron level

Some discussion of the nanoscale took place in Session I as follows:

David Williams	And then finally, some aspects of nanotechnology. This I am sure is going to be discussed in several sections. Way back in one of my first slides I referred to some general terms, and I put in there, nanoscale. A nanoscale will appear in almost any definition associated with nanotechnology. I know there's at least one person in the room who may disagree with me here, but that is what is part of this meeting is all about. Most organizations, scientific organizations, I say especially those in Europe, but not only in Europe, will define the nanoscale as being of around 100 nanometers or less. That is not arbitrary, it is because we have the effects of surface area to volume ratio and the fact that below 100 nanometers, you have quantum effects.
David Williams	When I was editing Biomaterials, I would never allow anybody who said that we have particles of 990 nanometers as being nanoscale. That is not nanoscale, that is slightly sub-micron to me. So we will bear that in mind.
David Williams	So nanotechnology: "the design, characterization, production, and application of structures, devices and systems, by controlling shape and size at the nanoscale." And then "nanomaterial." To me, the word nanomaterial is an absolute nonsense. What can a nanomaterial be? Many people use it, we have to recognize it is there, so we can't ignore it. I would like to say we should never use it, but it is there in common usage. So again, using other people's definitions, "any material with one or more external dimensions, or an internal structure which could exhibit novel characteristics compared to the same material without nanoscale features."
David Williams	To me, every material has a nanoscale feature. A grain boundary, a dislocation, or whatever. It is very difficult to determine what that means.
David Williams	And my last term, nanoparticle. And this has been a very difficult one. The definition should clarify dimensions. I give two here, or there could be three. One is "particle with one or more dimensions at the nanoscale." Or "particle with two or more dimensions at the nanoscale." You could add "particle with three dimensions at nanoscale." What are we the differences I am referring to here? If a three-dimensions are the nanoscale, you've essentially got a spheroid, which all dimension are 100 nanometers or less. If you have a nanorod or a whisker, then you have two dimensions at the nanoscale. If you have a plate, or platelet, you have one dimension

	at the nanoscale. Do we want to be inclusive of all these, or do we want to be specific?
Yuliang Zhao	I'm interested about the nanotechnology. The first point is that, I actually like the definitions most of them I agree with and as you look at that for nanomaterial and nanotechnology there are some different definitions from the United States and the UK and Asia countries. Actually, there are the terms, but for the biotechnology and the first is that the design for the nanotechnology. I am not sure this is for...just the definition for nanotechnology, just in biomaterial or in technology this first one. And the second is for the second one, we see that nanomaterials and one or more dimensions or an internal structure which could be compared to the same materials not at the nanoscale.
Yuliang Zhao	Actually, for most nanomaterials and some of them have different properties as we compare with the biomaterials but some of them will be different even at several hundred nanometers, five nanometers, or even larger but they have quite different properties. But some nanomaterial properties the size will go to several ten nanometers, ten nanometers because just the changes of the property. So in this case is such as that we just and that's the words and the compare to the same material result nanoscale features but tend into the same materials. For different materials, some changes properties where marginally at several ten nanometers but some of them several hundred nanometers so this is quite difficult to compare with the nanoscale.
Yuliang Zhao	The second one is nanoparticles with one or more dimension at the nanoscale, with the nanoparticles. But actually with nanoparticles the most important feature is the nanosurface. This is the difference. I suggest that we should include the nanosurfaces because most of the properties that are changing, the law of properties of collectivization comes from the unit surface structures or surface chemistries or surface electronics. So that property is clearer for definitions of nanoparticles. Thank you.
David Williams	I think you make some very good points there. The reason I have not mentioned surface area there is because you're absolutely right, it is the surface area to volume ratio which is very important for the properties of nanoparticles, but that is implied in the definition of nanoscale. That 100 nanometers or less. And if you look at the Royal Society, the Royal Academy of Engineering and the European Commission definitions, they make specific reference to the fact that below 100 nanometers, you have quantum effects, and the effects of the surface. So I am not sure we need to repeat that here when talking about nanoparticles. That is implicit in the nanoscale in my opinion.
Rena Bizios	Regarding the definition of the nanomaterial, what is your opinion in terms of nanostructures instead of nanomaterial, number one.

| | And number two, my experience has been that the biological, physiological environment is defined almost exclusively with surface and directions. Therefore, the bulk of the material, whether it is nano or any other scale, in my experience does not come into play, therefore I think that we have to maintain this particular distinction between the nanoscale features versus the materials which have the same chemical composition, but they have the whatever you call it, the other structures which are not nanoscale. |

Nicholas Peppas   The nanotechnology slide. The second part nanomaterial. I agree with you that it maybe doesn't make sense. But the reality all of us know, you know very well, that if you have two or three layers of material, the end-to-end distance and the configuration, the radius of gyration for polymer, may give it a totally different structure. For example, I have a polyvinyl alcohol, which all of us know is hydrophilic. But if I cast it next to a hydrophobic surface and if I oscillate only three layers which will make it nano level, it may show by your...hydrophobic characteristic, simply because the hydroxyl groups have flipped inside. Because they are in contact with a silicone. So is this your definition, your proposed definition? In the middle for nanomaterials?

Cato Laurencin   I just want to make a comment on the concept of nanotechnology and nanomaterials in the context of size. There has been a suggestion by a couple of people that we should be defining the nanoscale as that under a hundred nanometers. There are some areas in physics which I think that's appropriate. Feynman, 50 years ago when he first started talking about nanoscale and said there's plenty of room at the bottom, first looked at that range of under 100 nanometers. In the physics world, it is there. However, I think in the biological world, that scale really broadens a lot. So, if we think about the basic building block in terms of collagen, it is tropocollagen. Tropocollagen has a length scale of 300 nanometers. That's the building block: 300 nanometers. Many of us have worked in this area; we can see changes between 500 nanometers and 1200 nanometers in terms of cellular response, and we can actually - by changing the collagen fibril's diameter, fibril size - we can control a lot of the parameters around cell growth and phenotypic expression.

Cato Laurencin   In the physics range, yes. 30, 40 nanometers, go for it. In the range of biology, I believe that that scale is much broader. In fact, I think it starts at even a higher level in terms of the different areas. I want to make sure, in terms of our context of nano-size, that we're staying true to what is going on in terms of biology.

Editor's Note: These points are taken up in the Commentary and Summary Chapter that follows.

X

Commentary and summary

The complexity of the discussions at this conference confirmed that the formulation of scientifically valid definitions of terms used in a multi- and interdisciplinary field such as biomaterials science, that are both useful and understandable, is not a trivial issue. Several generic issues arose during these sessions which reinforced the inherent difficulty in achieving consensus; in most cases, there were no inherently right or wrong positions, and indeed it was difficult to maintain consistency across the spectrum of terms that were discussed. Nevertheless, considerable progress was made in confirming some existing definitions, making significant changes to previously established definitions and, especially, producing definitions (and, indeed, clarifying concepts) in areas of the science and applications of biomaterials that are very new, or only just emerging.

In this commentary, the more important of these generic issues are analyzed and then a summary of those definitions that achieved consensus is provided. It should be recalled that consensus means that 75% of those voting (exempting those who abstained) agreed with and supported the proposed definition. The status of provisional consensus was given to definitions that received over 50% of votes but not 75% or higher; in several situations, provisional consensus was achieved with newly emerging terms; this implies good support for the concept but suggests that refinement is required in the future.

A Generic Issues

(a) The Biomaterials Context

The first point here concerns the biomaterials context. In the introductory chapter to these proceedings, it was emphasized that biomaterials science is dependent on many individual disciplines, both technological and clinical, and we have to rely on the words, and their definitions, that primarily belong to these disciplines. It was not the intention to examine, dispute, or reinvent, any of these basic terms. It was considered important, however, to consider some well-known terms to see if any modifications were necessary to place them within the context of biomaterials science. Some delegates questioned why we were discussing definitions of clinical conditions, for example, stenosis, or why we were discussing established biological phenomena such as complement activation; the answers

Definitions of Biomaterials for the Twenty-First Century
DOI: https://doi.org/10.1016/B978-0-12-818291-8.00010-9

to both of these questions lay within the framework of the biomaterials context but, in reality, because so many terms had been placed on the provisional agenda for which there was insufficient time in the plenary sessions, few terms of questionable or marginal relevance were actually discussed.

(b) The Biomaterial—Medical Product Conundrum

At the time of the 1986 definitions conference, biomaterials were almost exclusively used in medical devices, including implantable medical devices and artificial organs. Today, biomaterials are used in very many more applications, including regenerative medicine, and drug and gene delivery. No attempt was made in the 2018 conference to delve into regulation-based definitions of medical products, but it is sometimes very difficult to separate out truly biomaterials-oriented scientific facts from issues that depend on the individual applications.

The definition of biocompatibility, agreed in 1986 and reconfirmed in 2018, is a good example of one that is biomaterials-related but does not differentiate between applications; this is probably why this contextual definition has stood the test of time but is also why it has limited usefulness since it does not inform the reader of how to design a biomaterial with better biocompatibility. Several times during discussions in Chengdu, this conundrum became very apparent, particularly with respect to blood compatibility and inflammation, which are both material and application dependent; this was the main reason why it was so hard to achieve consensus on these definitions.

It should also be noted that there was quite a difference between established terminology and innovative concepts. Several long-established terms generated quite antagonistic contributions, while some recently introduced technologies, such as "biochip" and "organoid" were far more readily accepted. This could well be due to the fact that the former, over decades of use, have become associated with well-entrenched views, while the latter generate interest and excitement without historical baggage.

(c) The Abuse of Words: Slang and Common Usage

Issues of slang words and the abuse of terminology surfaced on several occasions. Certain words, such as "smart material," "nanomaterial," and "material genome" make no sense scientifically. However, such terms are in widespread use, largely for marketing, legal, or grantsmanship reasons, and, as one delegate pointed out, purists have already lost the argument when we consider the use of "computer virus." Further comment on "nano" issues will be made later, but it is worth noting that the delegates largely agree with the avoidance of "smart" and "genome" with respect to biomaterials since these descriptors are clearly wrong, and agreed that slang terminology should not be encouraged.

One word needs a particular focus, that of "intelligent," as in "intelligent material" or "intelligent biomaterial." Several delegates expressed the view that this was no different to "smart" and should not be used; others took the other view that the use of this word was entirely acceptable. This is where common usage has to be taken into account. The concept of "intelligence" outside the animal kingdom, or indeed outside human experience according to some, is rather difficult to rationalize in terms of the usual connotation that intelligence has to encompass judgment and intuition. However, the essential equivalence of human intelligence and machine intelligence was being discussed nearly two hundred years ago as Babbage was working on his Difference Engine, the forerunner of the computer, when it was believed that the core of his technology, the ability to receive externally generated signals and the capacity to register and interpret signals, was encompassed by "intelligence." The massive increase in interest and application of artificial intelligence enhances this view that "intelligence" is now acceptable, provided that we bear in mind the fundamental difference between "artificial" or "machine" intelligence and natural intelligence.

(d) Drugs and Therapeutic Agents

The use of biomaterials as carriers to deliver substances to the body in a manner that is different to conventional oral or parenteral routes presented some difficulties with respect to the nature of these substances and the role of the nature of these substances on the characteristics of the delivery process. Initially this field involved drugs, but now we have to consider genes, vaccines, and diagnostic agents. We also have to encompass small molecules and proteins, and delivery times ranging from a few seconds up to several months, the essential features involving the control over the delivery kinetics and the route by which the substance gets to the target location. Generally, the definitions agreed in the conference did not differentiate between different characteristics of these substances. One issue that arose in several places was the difference between a drug and a therapeutic agent. Ideally a drug, or pharmaceutical agent, is discussed in terms of its chemistry, while therapeutic agent is discussed in terms of the effect on the patient. Although some delegates suggested that differences could be based on molecular size, this was not a consistent view, and in the definitions given, no attempt has been made to discriminate between drugs and therapeutic agents.

(e) The Nanoscale

It had been planned to discuss some nanotechnology-related terms such as "nanomaterial" and "nanoparticle," but time did not permit this. However, some reference was made to the concept of the "nanoscale" and an important point was raised. The conference confirmed that the scientific community's definition of the nanoscale as "having one or more dimensions of the order of 100 nm or less" is correct, primarily because of the significant increase in effects of the surface area to volume ratio of particles at these dimensions, and the contribution of quantum effects at even smaller dimensions.[1] However, the conference recognized that these effects were largely attributed to physical phenomena, and that such a limit was not so relevant with biological phenomena.[2] The conference, therefore, while not diminishing in any way the physical limitation of approximately 100 nm for the nanoscale, urged that the biomaterials (and possibly broader biotechnology/biomedical engineering) community uses a more flexible approach when considering the nanoscale in

[1] Nanoscience and nanotechnologies: opportunities and uncertainties, The Royal Society and Royal Academy of Engineering (UK), 29th July 2004.

[2] Safinya CR et al., Nanoscale assembly in biological systems: from neuronal cytoskeletal proteins to curvature stabilizing lipids, Adv. Mater, 2011;23(20):doi:10.1002/adma.201004647.

biological systems. Such flexibility, of course, has to be scientifically sound and not used for marketing, regulatory, or litigation reasons.

One final comment here concerns the word "nanomaterial." The conference recognized that this word was now in very common use, and cannot be ignored, even though it is scientifically irrelevant. The conference did not endorse any definition of this word.

B Terms With Definitions That Achieved Consensus and Which Supported or Slightly Modified Existing Definitions

We first summarize those definitions that confirmed, or essentially confirmed, existing definitions. The figures in brackets after the term provide the percentage of YES votes)

Biocompatibility (97.9%)

"The ability of a material to perform with an appropriate host response in a specific application"

Bioceramic, synonymous with Ceramic Biomaterial (90.9%)

"Any ceramic, glass or glass-ceramic that is used as a biomaterial"

Hydrogel (95.4%)

"A physically or chemically cross-linked polymer, swollen in water or biological fluids"

Thrombogenicity (93.9%)

"The tendency of a material in contact with blood to form a thrombus"

Biodegradation (90%)

"Breakdown of a material mediated within a biological system"

Implant (84.1%)

"A medical device made from one or more biomaterials that is intentionally placed, either totally or partially, within the body"

Percutaneous and Transcutaneous (100% Taken together)

Percutaneous "Taking place through the skin, involving disruption of the skin"

Transcutaneous "Penetrating, entering or passing through the intact skin"

Bioprosthesis (95.7%)

"Implantable prosthesis that consists totally or substantially of non-viable, human or animal donor tissue"

Stent (100%)

"A tubular support placed in a blood vessel, canal or duct to aid healing, or prevent or relieve an obstruction or stenosis"

Drug Delivery (93.1%)

"Delivery and/or release of therapeutic and/or diagnostic agents"

Controlled Release (95.7%)

"Release of a solute, drug, diagnostic or therapeutic agent from a carrier, system, or device in a planned predictable manner"

Pulsatile Delivery (95.8%)

"Drug, therapeutic or diagnostic agent delivery through a formulation that can produce successive steps of high and low rates"

Zero-order Release (95.8%)

"Release of a therapeutic agent at a constant rate over time"

C Terms With Definitions That Achieved Consensus and Which Significantly Modified Existing Definitions

Biomaterial, synonymous with Biomedical Material (91.1%)
"A material designed to take a form that can direct, through interactions with living systems, the course of any therapeutic or diagnostic procedure"
Regeneration (94%)
"Synthesis, renewal or growth of new functional tissue for use where tissue has failed due to aging or disease, or has been lost through injury, or because of congenital deficiency"
Regenerative Medicine (95.6%)
"Therapies that treat disease, congenital conditions or injury by the regeneration of functional tissue or organ structures"
Tissue Engineering (88.8%)
"The use of cells, biomaterials and suitable molecular or physical factors, alone or in combination, to repair or replace tissue to improve clinical outcomes"
Scaffold (80.9%)
"A biomaterial structure that serves as a substrate and guide for tissue repair and regeneration"

D Terms With Definitions That Achieved Consensus and Which Underpin Emerging Technologies

Responsive Biomaterial (97.8%)
"A biomaterial whose physical state is designed to have a predictable response to external environmental conditions"
Tissue-Inducing Biomaterial (87.2%)
"A biomaterial designed to induce the regeneration of damaged or missing tissues or organs without the addition of cells and/or bioactive factors"
Mechanotransduction (93.9%)
"The processes by which cells sense mechanical stimuli and convert them to biochemical signals that elicit specific cellular responses"
Macrophage Phenotype (79.6%)
"The characteristic endocrine, exocrine, paracrine, and membrane functions of macrophages affecting the resolution of inflammation, repair and remodeling; there is a spectrum of distinct functional phenotypes in a stimuli dependent continuum, ranging in polarization states from pro-inflammatory M1 phenotype to anti-inflammatory M2 phenotype"
Myofibroblast (81.25%)
"Primary extracellular matrix - secreting cells, which contain alpha-smooth muscle actin, that are active during wound healing and fibrosis and are responsible for the contractility of scar tissue by modulation of matrix stiffness through focal adhesions; their

progenitors include resident fibroblasts, fibrocytes, pericytes and may also result from epithelial/endothelial to mesenchymal transition"

Decellularization (89.8%)

"The processing of tissues or organs to remove cells and cellular debris, with the aim of preserving biological activity and/or structural integrity of the extracellular matrix"

Recellularization (95.4%)

"The repopulation of decellularized tissues or organs by cells with the objective of ultimately reintroducing functional activity"

Biodegradable Metal (80.4%)

"A pure metal, alloy, or metal matrix composite that is intended to degrade in vivo"

Immunoisolation (93.5%)

"A strategy in which antigens that are present on an allograft or xenograft are prevented from coming into direct contact with the host immune system"

Biochip (100%)

"A miniaturized array or system for methodically and simultaneously measuring multiple biological or chemical properties for systematic diagnosis and detection"

Organ-on-a-chip (100%)

"Cell-culture models integrated into microfluidic devices to mimic the biological activity, dynamic biophysical environment, and/or biochemical functionalities of a given tissue or organ system"

Microphysiological System (97.8%)

"Interconnected tissues- or organs-on-a chip using human cells to support physiologically-relevant evaluations of complex interacting biological systems for drug screening and disease modeling"

Organoid (95.7%)

"Self-organized three-dimensional tissues that are typically derived from stem cells, and embedded in a matrix, and which mimic the key functional, structural and biological complexity of an organ"

Biomaterialomics (76.6%)

"Integration of computational tools, large databases and experimental techniques to explore the basic material elements and combine them to discover and design new biomaterials for medical products"

Bioink (89.1%)

"Cell-laden biomaterial that can be integrated into additive manufacturing processes to print 2D and 3D structures"

E Terms With Definitions That Achieved Provisional Consensus and Which Underpin Emerging Technologies

Biohybrid Material (73.5%)

"A biomaterial that is composed of both biological and synthetic components"

Regenerative Engineering (63.3%)

"The integration of advanced materials sciences, stem cell science, engineering, developmental biology and clinical translation for the regeneration of complex tissue and organ systems"

Whole Organ Engineering (55.6%)

"The engineering of replacement organs that results in the preservation of tissue type specific matrix in a 3D architecture that closely mimics the native tissue and seeks to provide organ-specific functionality"

Template (69.5%)

"Biomaterials-based construct of defined size, chemistry and architecture that controls the delivery of molecular and mechanical signals to target cells in tissue engineering processes"

Intracellular Delivery (66.7%)

"Delivery of drugs, therapeutic or diagnostic agents into specific cells"

Bio-click Reactions (71.4%)

"Processes involving orthogonal groups that react under near-biological conditions, yielding single, stable products, with either no or non-toxic byproducts, proceeding quickly in complex milieu, with high yield"

F Other Terms With Definitions That Achieved Consensus or Provisional Consensus Which Place Conventional Terms Into the Context of Biomaterials Science

Biopolymer (75.5%, Consensus)

"A polymer synthesized by living organisms"

Inflammation/Innate Immunity (71.7% Provisional Consensus)

"The response to injury and/or contact with biomaterials, involving a cascade of activation with blood cells and humoral factors, and both acute and chronic inflammation. In the case of implanted devices this may lead to resolution with fibrous capsule formation and remodeling; with ex vivo devices, this may lead to systemic effects"

Adaptive Acquired Immune System (83.3% Consensus)

"A system consisting of lymphocytes and their products, including antibodies; humeral immunity is mediated by B lymphocytes and their secreted immunoglobulins and cellular immunity is mediated by T lymphocytes including helper, cytotoxic and regulatory lymphocytes and natural killer cells"

Hypersensitivity Reaction (82.2% Consensus)

"Tissue injury acquired immune reaction produced by one of four mechanisms:

Type I – Immediate production of IgE antibody;
Type II – Antibody Mediated, production of IgG and/or IgM;
Type III – Immune Complex Mediated, deposition of antigen-antibody complexes with complement activation;
Type IV – Cell Mediated, activation of T lymphocytes"

Blood Compatibility (65.9% Provisional Consensus)

"The ability of a blood-contacting biomaterial to (1) avoid the formation of a thrombus by minimal activation of platelets and of blood coagulation, (2) minimize activation of the complement system and (3) minimize hemolysis"

Complement Activation (97.7% Consensus)

"A cascade of enzymatic reactions that when activated produce effector molecules involved in inflammation, cell adhesion, phagocytosis and cell lysis"

Prosthesis (72.3% Provisional Consensus)

"Device that replaces or augments a part of the body"

Stenosis (85.1% Consensus)

"A narrowing or constriction of a tubular organ or structure"

Therapeutic Agent (97.6% Consensus)

"A substance used to treat a disease or other medical condition"

Provisional list of terms to be discussed and examples of possible definitions

Members of the Executive Committee who met in Chengdu in January 2018 were provided with a provisional list of terms that could be discussed and defined at the Consensus Conference. This list was amended during the January meeting and refined over the following months. The provisional list, along with suggestions of the Editor, David Williams, for possible definitions, is provided in this Annex. It is emphasized that the Plenary Speaker for each session was free to add to or delete the suggested terms and were under no obligation to use any of the suggested definitions. In some cases, a citation has been given for a suggested definition; in most cases the suggestion(s) have been derived from an analysis of definitions in major dictionaries and reference works and adapted or modified to suit the context of the 2018 consensus conference.

General Biomaterials; Plenary Speaker David Williams

Biomaterial

1. A non-viable material used in a medical device, intended to interact with biological systems; *Definition that achieved consensus in Chester 1986*
2. Any matter, surface, or construct that interacts with biological systems[1]
3. A material intended to interface with biological systems to evaluate, treat, augment or replace any tissue, organ or function of the body[4]

[1] National Institute of Biomedical Imaging and Bioengineering (USA:NIH)

4. A substance that has been engineered to take a form which, alone or part a complex system, is used to direct, by control of interactions with components of living systems, the course of any therapeutic or diagnostic procedure, in human or veterinary medicine[3]

Biomedical Material

A material intended to interface with biological systems to evaluate, treat, augment or replace any tissue, organ or function of the body[4]

Bioceramic

Any ceramic, glass or glass-ceramic that is used as a biomaterial

Biopolymer

1. Naturally occurring long-chain molecules
2. A polymeric substance formed in a biological system
3. Polymer synthesized by living organisms

Polymeric Biomaterial (synonymous with Biomedical Polymer)

Any polymeric material, either natural or synthetic, that is used as a biomaterial

Metallic Biomaterial

Any metallic material that is used as a biomaterial

Biodegradation

1. Gradual breakdown of a material mediated by specific biological activity; *Definition that achieved provisional consensus in Chester 1986*
2. Breakdown of a material mediated by a biological system, *Refined version of (1) above, that eliminates reference to "gradual" and "specific"*
3. The process by which organic substances are decomposed by micro-organisms (mainly aerobic bacteria) into simpler substances such as carbon dioxide, water and ammonia[2]

Biodegradable Polymer

A polymer which degrades as a result of the action of naturally occurring active species where the rate of degradation takes place in a specified time period comparable to existing natural processes

Biostability

1. Capacity of a material to resist chemical or structural degradation within a biological environment.[4] Note that this is a relative term since all materials undergo some change over time in biological environments. In practice, it refers to situations where there are no clinical consequences associated with such change.
2. Condition in which a material resists chemical and/or structural changes within a biological environment that have any clinical consequences. *Modification of (1) above.*

[2] OECD: Glossary of Statistical Terms

Bioresorption

1. Process of removal by cellular activity and /or dissolution of a material in a biological environment; *Definition that achieved provisional consensus in Chester 1986*
2. The breakdown of a structure within a biological environment and the consequent assimilation of resulting components into that environment

Bioabsorption

Process whereby substances are absorbed by the tissues and organs in a living system

Biomimesis (Synonymous with Biomimicry)

Utilization of knowledge of the formation, structure or function of biologically produced substances or of biological processes, for the purpose of designing similar substances or processes by artificial means

Bioinspired Material

Synthetic material whose structure, properties or function mimics those of natural materials or living matter

Medical Device

1. An instrument, apparatus, implement, machine, contrivance, in vitro reagent, or other similar or related article, including any component, part or accessory, which is intended for use in the diagnosis of disease or other conditions, or in the cure, mitigation, treatment or prevention of disease, in man. *Definition that achieved consensus in Chester 1986*
2. Any health care product that is intended for the diagnosis, prevention, or treatment of disease or injury and does not primarily work by effecting a chemical change in the body

Nanotechnology

The design, characterization, production and application of structures, devices and systems by controlling shape and size at the nanoscale

Nanomaterial

Material with one or more external dimensions, or an internal structure, which could exhibit novel characteristics compared to the same material without nanoscale features

Nanoparticle

1. Particle with one or more dimensions at the nanoscale
2. Particle with two or more dimensions at the nanoscale

Biocompatibility, Plenary Speaker James Anderson

Biocompatibility

The ability of a material to perform with an appropriate host response in a specific application; *Definition that achieved consensus in Chester 1986*

Innate Immunity

An immunological subsystem that provides the first line of defense against infection or foreign body-induced responses, in a non-specific manner, independent of antigens

Adaptive Immunity (synonymous with Acquired Immunity)

An immunological subsystem, characterized by memory, that provides protection from a pathogen or toxin, being mediated by B and T cells and highly specific to a given antigen

Hypersensitivity

An abnormal sensitivity to an allergen, drug or other agent, associated with an exaggerated immune response

Bioactivity

A phenomenon by which a biomaterial elicits or modulates biological activity

Bioactive Material

A material which has been designed to induce specific biological activity: *Definition that achieved consensus in Chester 1986*

Blood Compatibility

Note that the use of this term was deprecated at the Chester 1996 Conference since it was too general.

Thrombogenicity

The property of a material which induces and / or promotes the formation of a thrombus; *Definition that achieved consensus in Chester 1986*

Carcinogenicity

Ability or tendency to produce cancer.[4] *Note that although tumorigenicity is a better term technically since all cancers involve tumors but not all involve carcinomas, carcinogenicity is the preferred term because of greater common use*

Tumorigenic

Capable of producing a tumor

Complement Activation

Process in which serum proteins of the complement system are involved in sequential activation by antibody-antigen complexes, cell walls or biomaterial surfaces, that produces effector molecules involved in inflammation, phagocytosis and other biological responses

Cell Adhesion

Process by which cells form contacts with each other, with their natural substratum of foreign surfaces through specific protein complexes

Cell Adhesion Molecule

Any of various molecules that exist on cell surfaces that are capable of attachment to molecules on other cells, on their natural substratum, other extracellular substances or foreign material surfaces

Inflammation

A localized tissue reaction, involving both cellular and humoral components, in response to infection, irritation of injury

Granulation

Reparative connective tissue that consists of new capillaries in an edematous environment of fibroblasts, myofibroblasts, inflammatory cells and cellular debris

Damage Associated Molecular Patterns

1. Endogenous molecules that are released into the extracellular space under conditions of activation, cellular stress, or tissue damage
2. An endogenous and heterogeneous group of molecules that warn the immune system of tissue damage and exhibit varying molecular characteristics, locations, and functions

Inflammasome

1. A multiprotein intracellular complex that detects pathogenic microorganisms and sterile stressors and that activates the highly pro-inflammatory cytokines IL-1b and IL-18
2. A multiprotein cytoplasmic complex which activates one or more caspases, leading to the processing and secretion of pro-inflammatory cytokines

Mechanotransduction

1. The processes by which cells sense mechanical stimuli and convert them to biochemical signals that elicit specific cellular responses
2. The molecular and cellular processes that are involved with the conversion of mechanical stimuli into biochemical signals[3]

---

[3] Williams DF, Biocompatibility pathways: Biomaterials-induced sterile inflammation, mechanotransduction, and principles of biocompatibility control, *ACS Biomaterials Sci Eng*, 2017, 3(1), 2-35.

Implantable and Interventional Devices; Plenary Speaker Jiang Chang

Implant (synonymous with Implantable Device)

A medical device made from one or more biomaterials that is intentionally placed within the body, either totally or partially buried beneath an epithelial surface; *Definition that achieved consensus in Chester 1986*

Percutaneous

Taking place through the skin, involving disruption of the skin; *Note 'per' and 'trans' both could mean 'through' or 'across'. Convention and usage now determines that with respect to skin, 'per' implies that passage through the skin involves some degree of physical penetration whereas 'trans implies the skin remains intact*

Transcutaneous

Penetrating, entering, or passing through the intact skin; *Note 'per' and 'trans' both could mean 'through' or 'across'. Convention and usage now determines that with respect to skin, 'per' implies that passage through the skin involves some degree of physical penetration whereas 'trans implies the skin remains intact*

Bioprosthesis

Implantable prosthesis that consists totally or substantially of non-viable, treated, donor tissue, *Definition that achieved consensus in Chester 1986*

Stenosis

Narrowing or contraction of a duct or canal

Restenosis

The reoccurrence of stenosis after it has been treated with apparent success

Stent

1. A tubular support placed temporarily inside a blood vessel, canal, or duct to aid healing or relieve an obstruction
2. A short narrow metal or plastic tube often in the form of a mesh that is inserted into the lumen of an anatomical vessel (such as an artery or a bile duct), especially to keep a previously blocked passageway open
3. An intravascular stent is a synthetic tubular structure intended for permanent implant in native or graft vasculature. The stent is designed to provide mechanical radial support after deployment; this support is meant to enhance vessel patency over the life of the device. Once the stent reaches the intended location, it is expanded by a balloon or self-expanding mechanisms defined below[4]

[4] US Food and Drug Administration

Transcatheter

Performed through the lumen of a catheter

Extracorporeal Circulation

1. Maintenance of blood circulation by means of pumps located outside of the body, with blood fed through catheters advanced in an appropriate blood vessel and returning to the body to another blood vessel
2. The circulation of blood outside of the body through a machine that temporarily assumes an organ's functions

Implant-related Infection

A host immune response to one or more microbial pathogens on an indwelling implant

Catheter-related Infection

A host immune response to one or more microbial pathogens associated with a catheter, diagnosed by both the presence of clinical manifestations of infection and the evidence of colonization of the catheter tip by microorganisms

Surgical Mesh

A mesh that may be implanted to support tissue or organs

Bridge – to – Transplant

The concept of using any organ or surrogate device to stabilize a patient before the definitive transplantation of a matched organ

Drugs and Genes; Plenary Speaker Nicholas Peppas

Drug Delivery System

1. Any multi-component device that has the intended function of delivering a drug to a patient in a known and controlled manner[4]
2. Engineered technologies for the targeted delivery and/or controlled release of therapeutic agents[7]

Targeted Drug Delivery

Process by which a drug is delivered to the site of action without it exerting any pharmacological effect elsewhere[4]

Drug Carrier

Any device or material used to control the delivery of a drug to tissues or cells

Liposome

A spherical artificial vesicle composed of one or more concentric phospholipid bilayers

Protein Therapeutic Agent (synonymous with Therapeutic Protein)

Polypeptides, used as drugs, whose active components are derived from a biological source and are produced in human or animal cells or in microorganisms[10]

Drug Elution

The transfer of a drug that is contained within, or adsorbed on, a biomaterial into surrounding biological environment

Theranostics

A personalized medicine approach that combines specific targeted therapy based on specific targeted diagnostic tests

Theranostic Agent

1. A biomaterial that combines diagnostic and therapeutic capabilities within a single agent
2. A product that incorporates both a drug delivery mechanism and an imaging / diagnostic agent[5]

Gene Therapy

1. The transplantation of genes into human cells in order to cure a disease caused by a genetic defect
2. The replacement or alteration of defective genes in order to prevent the occurrence of inherited diseases
3. The administration of genetic material to modify or manipulate the expression of a gene product or to alter the biological properties of living cells for therapeutic use[10]

Non-viral Gene Vector

A product or system, other than a virus-based agent, which contains or consists of a recombinant nucleic acid that is administered to living species in order to regulate, repair, replace, add to or delete a genetic sequence

Regenerative Medicine; Plenary Speaker William Wagner

Regeneration

1. Synthesis of new, natural tissue at the site of a tissue (one cell type) or organ (more than one cell type) which either has been lost due to injury or has failed due to a chronic injury[4]
2. The reactivation of development in later life to restore missing tissues
3. The restoration or new growth by an organism of tissues that have been lost

---

[5] Williams D F, *Essential Biomaterials Science*, Cambridge University Press, 2014

Regenerative Medicine

Therapies that treat disease and injury by the regeneration of functional tissue or organ structures[11]

Tissue Engineering

1. The creation of new tissue for the therapeutic reconstruction of the human body, by the deliberate and controlled stimulation of selected target cells through a systematic combination of molecular and mechanical signals[6]
2. The use of a combination of cells, engineering materials, and suitable biochemical factors to improve or replace biological functions in an effort to improve clinical procedures for the repair of damaged tissues and organs[7]

Cell Therapy

The process of introducing new cells into a tissue in order to treat disease[11]

Self-Assembly

1. The autonomous organization of components into patterns or structures without human intervention[8]
2. The autonomous organization of components into patterns or structures without management from outside sources

Reanimation

No definition offered

Bioink

A hydrogel biomaterial that can be extruded through a printing nozzle, maintaining shape fidelity after deposition, and providing a 3D environment with biologically relevant chemical and physical signals that mimic the natural extracellular matrix environment to support cell proliferation and differentiation

Scaffold

A porous structure which serves as a substrate and guide for tissue regeneration[4]

Template

Biomaterials-based construct of defined size, chemistry and architecture that controls the delivery of molecular and mechanical signals to target cells in tissue engineering processes[9]

---

[6] Williams DF, To engineer is to create; the link between engineering and regeneration, *Trends in Biotechnology* 2006;24(1):4-8.

[7] www.regenerativemedicine.net

[8] Whitesides GM & Grzybowski B, Self-assembly at all scales, *Science* 2002;295:2418.

[9] Williams DF, The biomaterials conundrum in tissue engineering, *Tissue Engineering*, Part A, 2014;20:1129-31.

Whole Organ Engineering

The engineering of replacement organs by the decellularization and subsequent recellularization of donor organs, that results in the preservation of tissue type specific matrix in a 3D architecture that closely mimics the native tissue and maintains the natural vasculature network

Tissue Integration

The functional incorporation of engineered tissue into a host

Tissue Equivalent

A product that is intended to replace or augment natural tissue and which has properties that are analogous to those of that tissue

Immunoprotection

Protection against the effects of an antigen

Immunoisolation

An immunological strategy in which non-self antigens that are present on an allograft or xenograft are prevented from coming into contact with the host immune system

Provisional Matrix

1. An open and loosely organized ECM present in both developmental and diseased tissue
2. A matrix that consists of fibrin, produced by activation of the coagulative and thrombosis systems, and inflammatory products, released by the complement system, activated platelets, inflammatory cells, and endothelial cells in response to a biomaterial

Emerging Biomaterials and Technologies; Plenary Speaker Kristi Anseth

Biochip

1. A miniaturized laboratory capable of performing thousands of simultaneous biochemical reactions
2. A hypothetical computer logic circuit or storage device in which the physical or chemical properties of large biological molecules are used to process information
3. An array of miniaturized chemical or biological test sites arranged on a substrate so that many tests can be performed simultaneously

Organ − on − a − Chip

A multi-channel, microfluidic device that contains cultured human cells within a controlled microenvironment to recapitulate the molecular, structural and physical characteristics of a given organ system

Bioimaging

The imaging of biological materials, structures, systems or processes.

Functional Imaging

Imaging modalities directed at the evaluation of activity and function of tissues or organs

Surface Topography

Delineation of the natural and artificial features of an area of a surface[4]

Surface Patterning

The deliberate, regular and spatially-controlled modification of surfaces through physical, chemical or biological means in order to enhance specific properties and performance

Biomaterials Genome

No definition offered

Immunomodulation

Adjustment of the immune response to a desired level

Bioartificial Organ

1. A product intended to repair, replace or augment tissues or organs that is derived from a combination of cells, biomolecules and biomaterials[4]
2. A device in which components of living tissues are embedded within biomaterial scaffolds to enable it to perform complex biochemical functions of a specified organ

Bioprinting

The use of 3D printing technology with biomaterials that incorporates viable cells in order to construct functional living tissue

Biosensor

A device used to detect the presence or concentration of a biological analyte

Thermogel

A substance that exhibits a sol-gel transition under the influence of heat

Microfluidics

The science of microminiaturized devices containing chambers and tunnels through which fluids flow in a controlled manner

Point-of-Care Devices

Devices used to obtain diagnostic results while with the patient or close to the patient

The Chengdu Declaration

The Chengdu Declaration of Definitions in Biomaterials Science

Biomaterials science emerged as an important discipline in the 1960s and evolved rapidly to a point where it was having a significant impact in healthcare technologies, especially involving implantable medical devices. As often happens with emerging fields, a plethora of terms and phrases were introduced into the literature to describe new phenomena and devices, often with a great deal of confusion over their meaning. Some of them were words that had been derived within an established area but were now being used in the biomaterials context with a different meaning. In other situations, there was a clear need for a new word to describe a process or object, where there was no acceptable existing word, but the introduction of the descriptive word or phrase did not follow etymological reasoning, or indeed, common sense. Part of the problem lay within the multi- and inter-disciplinary nature of the subject, as pathologists tried to describe corrosion mechanisms within metallic devices and metallurgists tried to describe inflammatory responses.

Whatever the cause of the laxity of definitions and of their undisciplined use, the results were the same; confusion about the subject under discussion, ambiguity in the literature and dangerous or misleading uncertainties in the promulgation of knowledge. Research, education and clinical uses all suffered. It was for this reason that the European Society for Biomaterials convened a consensus conference, in Chester, UK, in 1986, to discuss this terminology and to produce a series of recommended definitions. The proceedings were published in 1987[1]. In order for a definition to achieve a consensus, it had to be approved by at least 75% of those present.

Some of the definitions that achieved consensus have stood the test of time and are still widely used today. Many others became out-of-date quite quickly, as scientific understanding changed, and far more applications of biomaterials technology were introduced

---

[1] Williams DF (Ed), *Definitions in Biomaterials*, Progress in Biomedical Engineering, Vol 4, Elsevier, Amsterdam, 1987.

into clinical practice. It became obvious that a new look at biomaterials definitions was essential and that, with the enhanced globalization of this field, a broader international viewpoint would be preferable.

Accordingly, in June 2018, a new consensus conference was convened in Chengdu, Sichuan Province of the People's Republic of China, under the auspices of the International Union of Societies of Biomaterials Science and Engineering (IUSBSE). Essentially the same rules for achieving consensus that were applied in 1986 were adopted for 2018. The proceedings are again being published by Elsevier[2].

Approximately 50 terms were discussed. The terms covered included a selection of those discussed in Chester, some of which were confirmed as still being correct, others being modified or replaced. The discussions incorporated aspects of regenerative medicine, drug, gene and vaccine delivery and diagnostic biomaterials as well as implantable and interventional devices, with an emphasis on those clinical applications that have been emerging at the forefront of medical technology in the twenty-first century.

A few of the key definitions that achieved consensus were "responsive biomaterial", "tissue-inducing biomaterial", "regenerative medicine", "organoid", "biochip", "biomaterialomics" and "biocompatibility"

The delegates at the conference were of the unanimous view that the recommendations concerning these definitions of crucial scientific and clinical terms should be widely disseminated since they underpin the successful translation of new technologies to patient care and wellbeing.

Accordingly, the delegates, through this **Chengdu Declaration of Definitions in Biomaterials Science** draw the attention of the whole of the biomaterials science community, and especially journal editors and their editorial board and reviewers, to the importance of adhering to these basic principles of terminology.

Conference Chair
Xingdong Zhang, Sichuan University, Chengdu, China

Editors
Xingdong Zhang, Sichuan University, Chengdu, China
David Williams, Wake Forest Institute of Regenerative Medicine, Winston-Salem, USA

Executive Committee
James Anderson, Case Western Reserve University, Cleveland, USA
Kristi Anseth, University of Colorado at Boulder, Boulder, USA
Xiaobing Fu, General Hospital of PLA, Beijing, China
Kazunori Kataoka, University of Tokyo, Tokyo, Japan
Cato Laurencin, University of Connecticut, Hartford, USA
Keith McLean, CSIRO, Melbourne, Australia
Nicholas Peppas, University of Texas at Austin, Austin, USA
David Williams, Wake Forest Institute of Regenerative Medicine, Winston-Salem, USA
Xingdong Zhang, Sichuan University, Chengdu, China

---

[2] Zhang XD and Williams DF (Ed), Definitions of Biomaterials for the Twenty-First Century, Elsevier, 2018.

Plenary Speakers
James Anderson, Case Western Reserve University, USA
Kristi Anseth, University of Colorado at Boulder, Boulder, USA
Jiang Chang, Shanghai Institute of Ceramics, CAS, Shanghai, China
Nicholas Peppas, University of Texas at Austin, USA
William Wagner, University of Pittsburgh, USA
David Williams, Wake Forest Institute of Regenerative Medicine, Winston-Salem, USA

Delegates and Signatories of the Declaration
Hua Ai, Sichuan University, Chengdu, China
James Anderson, Case Western Reserve University, Cleveland, USA
Kristi Anseth, University of Colorado at Boulder, Boulder, USA
Iulian Antoniac, University Politehnica of Bucharest, Bucharest, Romania
Mário Barbosa, i3S/INEB, University of Porto, Porto, Portugal
Bikramjit Basu, Indian Institute of Sciences, Bangalore, India
Serena Best, University of Cambridge, London, UK
Ruggero Bettini, University of Parma, Parma, Italy
Deon Bezuidenhout, University of Cape Town, Cape Town, South Africa
Rena Bizios, University of Texas at San Antonio, San Antonio, USA
John Brash, McMaster University, Hamilton, Canada
Yilin Cao, Shanghai Jiao Tong University, Shanghai, China
Jiang Chang, Shanghai Institute of Ceramics, CAS, Shanghai, China
Guoping Chen, National Institute for Materials Science, Tsukuba, Japan
Elizabeth Cosgriff-Hernandez, University of Texas at Austin, Austin, USA
Arthur Coury, Northeastern University, Boston, USA
Jiandong Ding, Fudan University, Shanghai, China
Xiaobing Fu, General Hospital of PLA, Beijing, China
Andrés García, Georgia Institute of Technology, Atlanta, USA
Brendan Harley, University of Illinois, Urbana, USA
Jian Ji, Zhejiang University, Hangzhou, China
Kazunori Kataoka, University of Tokyo, Tokyo, Japan
Joachim Kohn, Rutgers University, New Brunswick, USA
Cato Laurencin, University of Connecticut, Hartford, USA
Kam Leong, Columbia University, New York, USA
Jui-Che Lin, National Cheng Kung University, Taipei, China
Changsheng Liu, East China University of Science and Technology, Shanghai, China
Helen Lu, Columbia University, New York, USA
Peter Ma, University of Michigan, Ann Arbor, USA
Keith McLean, CSIRO, Melbourne, Australia
Ling Qin, Chinese University of Hong Kong, Hong Kong, China
Ki-Dong Park, Ajou University, Suwon, Korea
Nicholas Peppas, University of Texas at Austin, Austin, USA
Laura Poole-Warren, University of New South Wales, Sydney, Australia
Seeram Ramakrishna, National University of Singapore, Singapore
John Ramshaw, CSIRO, Melbourne, Australia

Rui Reis, University of Minho, Minho, Portugal
Carl Simon, NIST, Gaithersburg, USA
Wei Sun, Drexel University, Philadelphia, USA
Yasuhiko Tabata, Kyoto University, Kyoto, Japan
Madoka Takai, University of Tokyo, Tokyo, Japan
Timmie Topoleski, University of Maryland, Baltimore, USA
Maria J. Vicent, CIPF, Valencia, Spain
William Wagner, University of Pittsburgh, Pittsburgh, USA
Yingjun Wang, South China University of Technology, Guangzhou, China
Yunbing Wang, Sichuan University, Chengdu, China
David Williams, Wake Forest Institute of Regenerative Medicine, Winston-Salem, USA
Frank Witte, Charité-Universitätsmedizin Berlin, Germany
Tingfei Xi, Peking University, Beijing, China
Hanry Yu, National University of Singapore and A *Star, Singapore
Kai Zhang, Sichuan University, Chengdu, China
Xingdong Zhang, Sichuan University, Chengdu, China
Yuliang Zhao, National Center for Nanoscience and Technology, Beijing, China

Index